GIA'S IRIE KITCHEN

Caribbean and African Vegetarian Cuisine

GIA & KAYA

AuthorHouse™
1663 Liberty Drive, Suite 200
Bloomington, IN 47403
www.authorhouse.com
Phone: 1-800-839-8640

First published by AuthorHouse   6/1/2009

ISBN: 978-1-4389-1792-4 (sc)

Printed in the United States of America
Bloomington, Indiana

This book is printed on acid-free paper.

authorHOUSE®

ACKNOWLEDGEMENTS

If it was not for my daughter Kaya I may not have been able to write this book alone, give Thanks and praise. Her own wiliness to explore our food and its heritage. Special thanks to my dearest friend Empress Aminata for all her encouragement and help. And special thanks to Lenel for all her technical support and support

Without you all this may not have been possible.

INTRODUCTION

I wanted eating to be healthy for my family, with out being boring. Living in America with Caribbean roots that are of African origins. I put together vegetarian meals that are tradition and my own creations and twist. Family and friends look forward to special occasions and affairs. Involve children in meal planning and preparing the meals, the learning process is rewarding and educational they then want to eat because they prepared it.

There are different types of vegetarians;

Ovo-Lacto; No meat or fish little dairy and eggs

Lacto Vegetarian; No meat or fish little dairy, no eggs

Vegan; No meet, or fish no dairy, no eggs

Raw; UN cooked vegetables its natural source

In this book there are recipes to satisfy each type of vegans that are out of the ordinary that can be used for meal planning and side dishes.

INSIDE THE KITCHEN

MAIN DISHES AND SIDE DISHES

BREADS AND PIZZAS

SOUPS AND STEWS

DRINKS AND BEVERAGES

MENUS

APPETIZERS

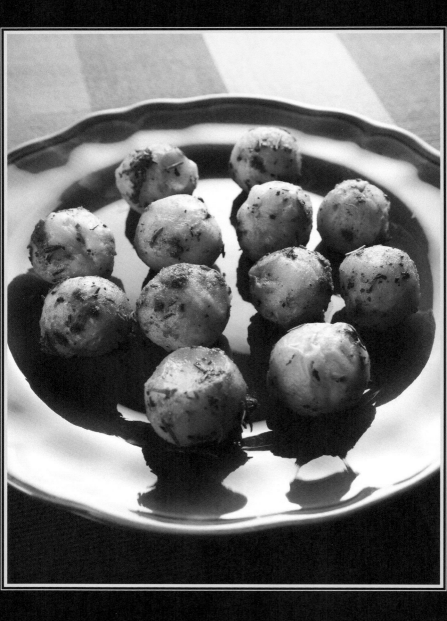

CORNY FRITTERS

- 10oz of corn
- 1/2 cup flour
- 1 cup water
- 1/4 cup butter
- 3 eggs
- 1tsp curry powder
- ½ tsp paprika

Mix flour, butter, curry powder, paprika, water, and 3 eggs.

Pour corn into batter and mix well. Drop by tablespoons into very hot oil.

Brown, drain on paper toweling. Serve with soca sauce

DABO KOLO
(Little Fried Snacks)

- 2 cups wheat or unbleached flour
- ½ tsp salt
- 2 T sugar
- ½ tsp cayenne pepper
- ¼ cup oil
- water

In a bowl mix flour, salt, sugar, cayenne, and oil. Knead together and add water. Spoonful by spoonful, to form stiff dough. Knead dough for 5 minutes longer. Tear off a piece the size of a golf ball. Roll it out with the palms of hands on a lightly floured board into a long strip ½ inch thick. Snip into ½ inch pieces with scissors. Spread about a handful of pieces on an ungreased frying pan. Cook over heat until uniformly light brown on all sides, stirring up once in a while as you go along. Continue until all are light brown.

FRIED EGGPLANT ROUNDS

- Eggplant (peeled and sliced)
- Cornmeal
- ¼ tsp dried parsley
- Peanut oil
- 1 egg
- Parmesan cheese (optional)

Peel and slice eggplant. In a bag mix Cornmeal and parsley, in a bowl beat egg add water if needed. Coat eggplant slices in egg. Then shake in bag until fully coated with cornmeal. Fry on both sides in peanut oil until golden brown and crispy. Immediately sprinkle with cheese once remove from pan.

GUNGO PEAS PATTY

- -salt for taste
- 1 clove of garlic
- ¼ cup wheat flour
- 1 ounce of margarine
- peanut oil for frying
- 1lb of green gungo peas
- 1 tablespoon of black pepper
- 2 medium sized chopped onion
- 1 scotch bonnet hot pepper

First soak and cook the peas until tender. Sauté the Onion, pepper and garlic in oil. Mash cooked peas and fold in sautéed seasonings. Add ¼ cup flour and form into patties. Fry in oil until lightly golden brown.

IRIE BITES

- 1 bag black eyed peas
- ½ cup chopped onions
- ½ cup chopped bell pepper
- scotch bonnet
- 2 cloves mashed garlic
- wheat flour
- bread crumbs
- oil for frying

Cook beans till soft mash and add in chopped onions, peppers garlic and chopped fine scotch bonnet form into 1 -2 inch balls roll in bread crumbs and wheat flour fry in oil till golden brown serve with flat bread or dips (see dips)

PLANTAIN SKINS

- 4-6 plantains
- peanut oil

Thoroughly wash plantain, and cut into thin slices with the skin on.

Fry in oil until golden crisp.

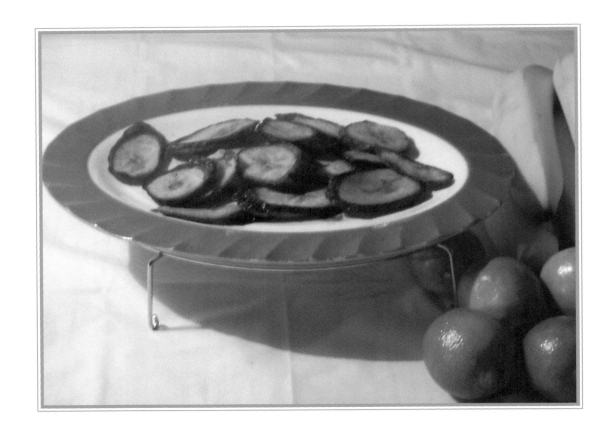

PRINCESS STICKS

- 10-12 bamboo skewers
- honey melon
- 20 strawberry
- 10-15 pineapple chunk
- papaya
- mango
- 5 banana
- 1T ground ginger
- 1T ground nutmeg
- 1tsp ground cinnamon
- ½ cup coconut milk(sweet)
- lemon juice
- lime juice
- orange juice

In a sauce pan warm sweet coconut milk and spices. Soak bamboo skewers for hour to prevent burning if going to grill fruit: Marinate fruit in the lime, orange and lemon juice to prevent fruit from turning brown.

Place fruit in even altering pieces on skewers suggest cutting melon, mango and papaya in squares can grill if desired pour warm sauce over fruit kabobs.

PUMPKIN FRITTERS

- 2 eggs
- 1 1/2 cup of flour
- 1/2 cup of milk or more
- 2 teaspoon of baking powder
- 1/4 teaspoon of chopped hot pepper
- 2 cup of pumpkin, cooked and crushed
- 1 tablespoon of melted butter or margarine

Sift together the flour, baking powder

And the salt. Beat the eggs until it's fluffy.

Next add the beaten eggs, hot pepper, melted margarine then the milk to dry

Ingredients and beat with a fork till its nice smooth.

Stir in crushed pumpkin, (batter should be of a dropping consistency) add more milk if desired. Drop by spoonfuls into preheated deep fat at 375 degrees F. Fry 4 to 5 min. Or until evenly browned.

RAGA, RAGA CHIPS

- 2 taro root← *yautia*
- 2 yellow yam
- 2 sweet potato
- 2 beets
- peanut oil for frying

Peel the yams and roots and slice with mandolin or sharp knife. Cut them in potato chip slices heat peanut oil and fry chips till crisp and lightly browned drain on paper can store in air tight container

RAS CUCUMBER CUPS

- 4-5 cucumber
- 1 cup chopped fresh spinach or callou
- ¼ cup chopped fine red onion
- ¼ cup chopped fine red bell pepper
- 1 tsp coriander
- 1 clove chopped and mashed garlic
- Yogurt or soy mayo
- Fresh mint

Chop onions and peppers small and fine suggest mashing with back of knife chop and mash garlic mix together with mayo or yogurt fold in spinach(or callou) and fresh chopped mint peel cucumber cut in to 1 inch half's use spoon or fruit spoon and scoop out centers add mixture in cups chill and serve

RASTA BABY LOGS

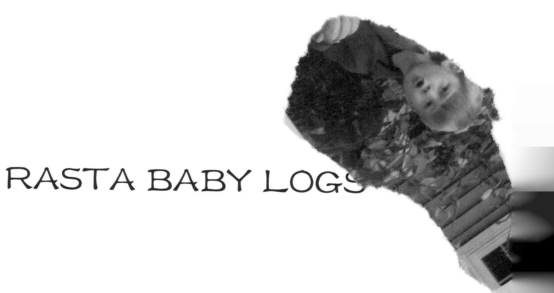

- 1 stalk celery
- 1 cup ground peanut paste
- ¼ cup honey
- 1 tsp ground nutmeg
- 1 tsp orange juice
- ¼ cup apple sauce

Cut celery into 3-4 inch pieces, Mix in a bowl peanut butter, honey, orange juice, apple sauce and fresh ground nutmeg spoon in to celery halves and chill great snack for kids.

ROASTED EGGPLANT

1 eggplant

1 jalapeño pepper

4 cloves garlic

1 onion

salt to taste

Make a slit in the eggplant and insert the garlic, and then cover the eggplant with oil. Slowly roast the eggplant in open fire until fully roasted. Remove the burnt skin and mash the eggplant in a bowl.

Slice onion and add to eggplant.

Heat 4 teaspoon of oil and add pepper and remainder of garlic. When it browns, mix with eggplant

SWEET POTATO FRIES

- 2 large sweet potatoes, peeled or unpeeled, cut into 4-inch long and 1/4 to 1/2-inch thick fries
- 2 tablespoons olive oil, or more as needed
- 1 teaspoon paprika
- 1/2 teaspoon chili powder
- 1/2 teaspoon ground coriander
- Coarse freshly ground black pepper, to taste

Preheat your oven to 450 degrees F. Line a baking sheet with aluminum foil and set aside.

Place the sweet potatoes in a large bowl and toss with olive oil until the sweet potatoes are coated. Add the paprika, chili powder, coriander, pepper; toss to distribute evenly.

Arrange the coated fries in a single layer on the prepared pan. Bake for 20 minutes on the lower rack until the sweet potatoes soften. Transfer the pan to the upper rack of the oven and bake 10 minutes longer, until fries are crispy. Serve with Avocado Dip.

VEGGIE STEAK FRIES

- 1 zucchini (cut into 3 inch sticks)
- 1 squash (cut into 3 inch sticks)
- 1 eggplant (cut into 3 inch sticks)
- 2 eggs
- ¼ cup milk
- 1 T onion powder
- 1 T garlic powder
- 1 T dried parsley
- 1 ½ cup panko bread crumbs
- 1 cup flour
- ½ cup parmesan cheese
- oil for frying

Thoroughly wash and cut all vegetables. In a bowl whisk eggs and milk, set aside. In another bowl mix Panko bread crumbs, parmesan cheese, garlic powder, onion powder and dried parsley. Heat oil for frying. Fry vegetables lightly until golden brown.

Dips and Sauces

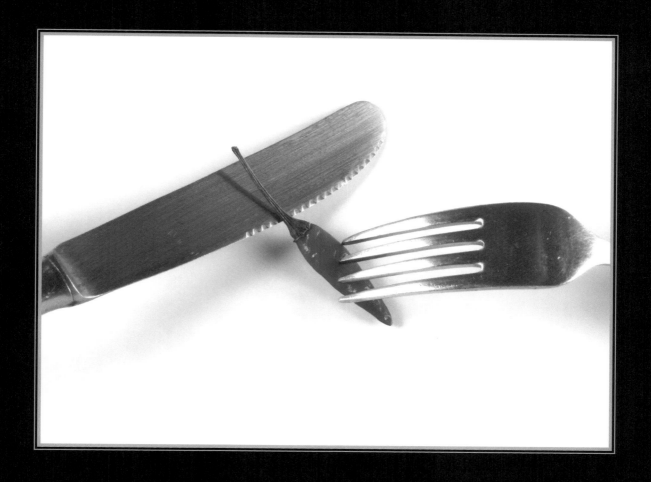

AVOCADO DIP

- 1 avocado
- 1/3 cup soy mayonnaise
- 1/3 cup cream cheese (optional)
- 1 jalapeno seeded and chopped.
- 2 scallions, white and light green part only, chopped
- 1 lime, juiced
- freshly ground black pepper

Place the avocado, soy mayonnaise, cream cheese, jalapeno, scallions, and lime juice into a blender or small food processor. Blend for 1 minute or until you have a smooth paste. Season with pepper to taste. Lime juice will prevent avocado from browning.

CHICKY PEA

- 2 cups cooked chick pea
- 1 cup cooked green pea
- 1 T grated onion
- 2 cloves garlic grated
- 1 T grated green bell pepper
- ¼ cup chopped seeded cucumber
- 2 T lemon juice
- 2 T lime juice
- ¼ cup extra virgin olive oil
- ¼ cup chopped cilantro
- ½ tsp chopped scotch bonnet

In a serving bowl combine the cooked peas and cucumber, add grated ingredients, whisk juice and oil, cilantro and chopped scotch bonnet together and fold in serve with bread or crackers.

CHILI LIME DIPPING SAUCE

- 1/3 cup sour cream
- 2 tablespoons mayonnaise
- 1 tablespoon lime juice (about 1/2 lime)
- 1/2 teaspoon chili powder
- zest of 1 lime

In a dipping bowl combine al ingredients. Let chill for several hours. Serve with favorite vegetables, breads, or crackers.

CURRY PASTE

- 6 tablespoons roasted coriander seeds
- 1 teaspoon roasted whole cloves
- 1 teaspoon ground turmeric
- 1 teaspoon roasted cumin seeds
- 1 teaspoon roasted fenugreek seeds
- 1 teaspoon roasted back peppercorns
- 1 teaspoon roasted mustard seeds
- 2 cloves garlic, chopped
- 1 large onion, chopped
- 1/2 scotch bonnet pepper chopped (Seeds and stem removed)
- Water as needed

Grind all of the ingredients into a paste with a mortar and pestle or puree in a food processor. Store in a jar and refrigerate.

ETHIOPIAN GREEN PEPPER RELISH

- large green bell pepper, very fresh
- medium garlic clove, coarsely chopped
- 1/8 teaspoon salt (to taste)
- jalapeno Chile, seeded and diced (optional)

Wash the bell pepper and coarsely chop. Put pepper, garlic and salt in the food processor fitted with a blade and scraping down the sides of the bowl repeatedly with a rubber spatula, process until rather smooth.

SWEET PEPPER & ROASTED GARLIC DIP

- 2 sweet red bell peppers
- 1/4 cup Roasted Garlic
- 1/4 cup extra-virgin olive oil
- 2 teaspoons fresh lemon juice
- 3 tablespoons chopped fresh basil leaves
- 1 teaspoon chopped fresh oregano leaves
- 1/4 teaspoon red pepper flakes, or to taste
- 2 teaspoons chopped fresh parsley leaves, garnish

Transfer the peppers and garlic to a food processor and process until smooth. With the machine running, slowly add 1/4 cup of the extra-virgin olive oil and lemon juice. Add the basil, oregano, red pepper flakes, and 1/4 teaspoon salt, and process until smooth. Adjust the seasoning, to taste. Transfer to a bowl and refrigerate for 1 hour.

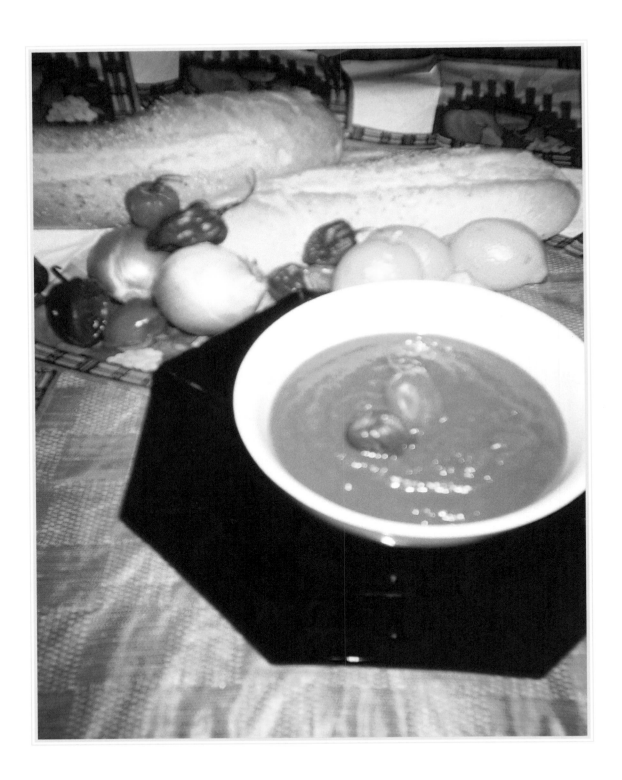

HARRISA
(ETHIOPIAN CONDIMENT)

- 4 (115 g) ounces dried chilies, soaked overnight
- cloves garlic, chopped
- 1/2 tablespoon ground coriander
- tablespoon ground caraway
- tablespoons mint, chopped
- tablespoons cilantro leaves, chopped
- tablespoon fresh parsley leaves, chopped
- 1/2 tablespoon rock salt
- tablespoon tomato puree
- tablespoon sugar
- tablespoons extra-virgin olive oil

Simmer the chilies for 2 minutes in a little water and soak for 1 hour and drain.

Blend with all the remaining ingredients in a food processor until smooth.

Pass through a strainer to remove any lurking chili seeds.

Put in a sterilized glass jar; dribble extra olive oil over the surface to create an airtight seal.

Keep refrigerated.

KWANZA CRANBERRY CHEESE DIP

- 8 oz cream cheese (soften)
- ¼ cup sour cream
- ½ cup dried cranberries (sun dried preferably)
- ½ tsp chives
- ½ tsp dried thyme
- orange zest

Mix all ingredients well. Serve with bread or crackers

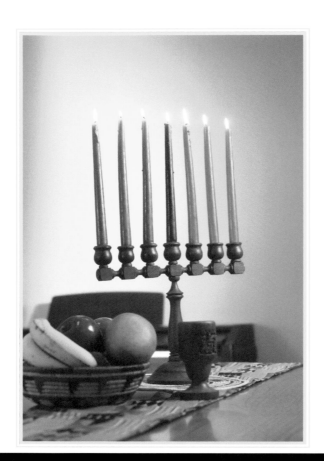

ONE LOVE DIP RED, GOLD, GREEN
(LAYERED DIP)

RED LENTIL LAYER:

- 1 bag red lentil (rinsed and soaked)
- 2 cloves garlic (grated)
- ¼ cup onion (grated)
- 1 tsp paprika
- 2 T lemon juice
- 1 tsp ground ginger
- 1 tsp cumin
- 1 tsp coriander

Combine all ingredients until lentils are tender. Set aside.

YELLOW SPLIT PEA LAYER:

- 1 bag yellow split pea (rinsed and soaked)
- ¼ cup yellow bell pepper (finely chopped)
- 2 cloves garlic (grated)
- ¼ cup onion (grated)
- ½ tsp turmeric
- ½ tsp curry powder

Combine all ingredients until peas are tender. Set aside.

WHOLE GREEN PEA LAYER

- 1 bag whole green peas (rinsed and soaked)
- 2 cloves garlic (grated)
- ¼ cup onion (grated)
- 1 tsp parsley
- ¼ tsp cayenne pepper

Combine all ingredients until peas tender. Set aside.

When all layers are done in a clear bowl lay red lentil layer on bottom. Then lay yellow split pea layer over the red lentil layer. Then lay green pea layer over yellow split pea layer. Serve warm or cold with Injera or flat bread.

SHEBA SAUCE

- Combine: 1 cup ketchup
- 1/4 Cup vinegar
- 1/2 Cup oil
- 1/2 Cup sweet white wine (muscatel or madeira)
- 1 Tsp. Worcestershire sauce
- 1 Tsp. Salt
- 1/4 Tsp. Black pepper
- Few drop tabasco sauce.
- Chopped tomatoes

Marinate the tomato mixture in the sauce. Serve in sauce dishes without lettuce or drain well and place in the center of the Injera

SKA SAUCE

- 2 cups kale
- 4-6 whole carrots
- 2 large tomatoes
- salt & pepper to taste if desired

Put all ingredients in juicer. Serve over favorite foods. Great on salads.

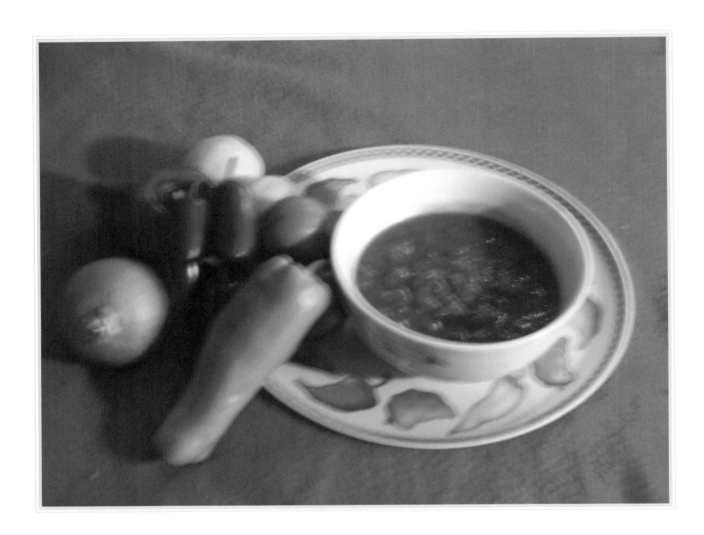

SOCA SAUCE

- 3 large ripe tomatoes
- 1 small onion
- ¼ cup red wine vinegar
- ½ tsp black pepper
- ¼ cup olive oil
- 1 T fresh parsley (chopped)
- ½ tsp red scotch bonnet pepper (minced)
- 2 large cloves garlic
- ½ cup water

With a box grater, grate tomatoes, onion, and garlic. In a bowl add remaining ingredients. Put in a blender and liquefy. Serve chilled over favorite food

SPICY CURRY DIP

- 1 cup sour cream
- 1 tsp curry powder
- ½ tsp cayenne pepper
- 1/2 T fresh lemon juice
- 1 Grated onion
- 1 clove garlic (minced)
- 1green bell pepper

Combine the sour cream, curry powder, cayenne pepper, lemon juice, and onion in a small bowl. Cover with plastic wrap and chill. Cut the bell pepper in half lengthwise, remove the core and seeds and serve the curry dip in a bowl topped with green bell pepper.

TROPICAL DRIED-FRUIT CHUTNEY

- pineapple juice
- 2 cinnamon sticks
- 1/2 cup of raisins
- 2 whole star anise
- 1 cup 1/2-inch dice dried
- -mango (about 4 1/2 ounces)
- 1 cup 1/2-inch dice dried
- -papaya (about 4 1/2 ounces)
- 1/2 cup 1/2-inch dice dried
- -pineapple (about 3 ounces)
- 1 vanilla bean, split lengthwise
- 3 tablespoons chopped fresh mint

In a heavy medium saucepan scrape the seeds from vanilla bean and add the bean, cinnamon sticks, and star anise.

Bring mixture to a simmer over medium heat.

Add all the dried fruits, return to simmer,

Occasionally stirring. To moisten chutney, mix in enough of the pineapple juice by tablespoonfuls.

Place into a bowl and cover then chill in the frigerator for 3 hours. Note: Chutney can be made 1 day ahead of time. Keep the Chutney refrigerated. Remove the vanilla bean, cinnamon sticks and star anise from chutney. Mix in mint

Main Dishes and Side Dishes

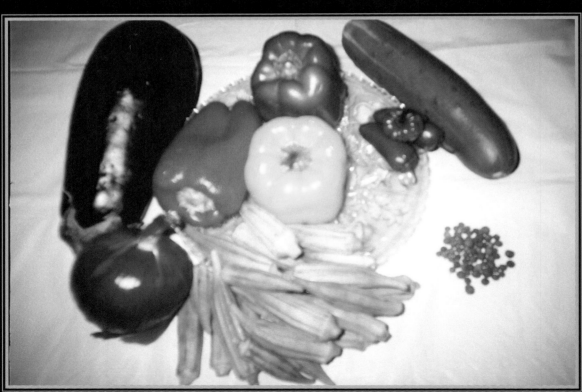

BAJAN BLACK BEAN CAKES WITH MANGO SALSA

MANGO SALSA:
- 2 cups mango (peeled & diced)
- ½ cup red bell pepper (diced)
- ¼ cup red onion (diced finely)
- 1 scotch bonnet pepper (minced)
- 2 T cilantro (coarsely chopped)
- 2 tsp ginger root (minced)
- 1 T lime juice

Combine all ingredients in a bowl. Set aside.

BLACK BEAN CAKES:
- 2 15oz cans black beans (rinsed)
- ¼ cup cilantro (chopped)
- ¼ cup red onion (chopped finely)
- 1 egg white (slightly beaten)
- 1 tsp ground cumin
- 1 tsp coriander
- ½ tsp ground allspice
- 1 clove garlic (minced)
- 1/8 tsp cayenne pepper
- 1/3 cup bread crumbs
- 1 T virgin olive oil
- Fresh chopped cilantro

Place the black beans in a large bowl and mash coarsely until they stick together. Add the cilantro, onion, egg whites, cumin, garlic, allspice and cayenne pepper. Mix until well blended. Divide the mixture into 8 equal parts. Shape into ½ inch thick patties. Coat the patties with bread crumbs. Fry bean cakes on both sides until golden brown. Serve with mango salsa. Garnish with cilantro.

BAKEY BEANS

- 1 bag pink beans
- ¼ cup chopped scallions
- ½ cup chopped yellow onion
- ½ cup chopped red bell pepper
- ½ cup chopped green bell pepper
- ¼ tsp cayenne pepper
- ¼ ground nutmeg
- 1T paprika
- pinch cinnamon
- 1 cup ketchup
- 2 T mustard
- water to cook beans
- 1 clove mashed garlic
- ½ cup brown sugar

Rinse and soak beans over night. Cook beans in water for several hours add onions, peppers, and seasonings in pan and sauté till tender add to cooking beans. An hour before done add brown sugar cook till beans are tender.

BANANA BOAT

- 1- 2banana leaf whole
- 2 cup cooked rice
- 1 cup cooked beans
- ¼ cup chopped onion
- ¼ cup chopped green pepper
- chopped fresh cilantro
- fresh thyme
- ½ cup seeded chopped tomato
- slice on bias green plantain

Soak banana leaf in water for half hour in center of banana leaf place rice beans and chopped veggies place plantain on top and fold in all sides. Roast, bake or grill.

BROWN STEWED VEGATABLES

- Cauliflower
- Broccoli
- Carrots
- onions
- Peppers
- Scallion
- Browning
- ½ cup Veggie broth
- pinch ketchup
- peanut oil

Cut veggies in stir fry size slices or chunks. Brown lightly in oil and simmer with veggie broth, pinch of ketchup and browning sauce cook till just tender.

CARIBBEAN GUISADO

Guisado is Caribbean style stew, Made through out the Caribbean. But in a vegan style.

- 2 cups of pumpkin, cubed
- 2 cups Celery root, chopped
- 2 cups Yucca, peeled and cubed
- 1 1/2 cups of chickpeas, cooked
- 2 cups potato, peeled and cubed
- 1 1/2 cups of pinto beans, cooked
- 8 Plum tomatoes, quartered lengthwise
- 2 medium Chayote squash cut in 2" pieces
- 1/4 cup of olive oil
- 1/4 teaspoon of salt
- 16 Whole garlic cloves
- 1 tablespoon of black pepper
- 3 tablespoons of ground cumin
- 1 teaspoon of hot pepper sauce
- 1/2 cup of fresh cilantro, chopped
- 4 large yellow onions, coarsely chopped

Preheat the oven to 300 degrees F. Combine all of the ingredients into a large roasting pan or casserole dish. Put in oven and cook, uncovered for at least 4 hours. Finally, the pumpkin, chayote and tomatoes will cook it down to a thick sauce. Stir every 30 minutes. Add more of the stock if needed.

CARRIBEAN CORN ON COB

- 6-8 whole ears of corn
- 2 cloves whole garlic
- 1 T garlic powder
- 4T dried thyme twigs
- 1 T paprika
- 1 T ground ginger
- 2 scotch bonnets
- 2 T curry powder
- ¼ cup ghee or butter

Par boil corn till just slightly done. In a sauce pan make butter sauce with dried seasonings and herbs and scotch bonnet once butter is saucy add corn and let finish cook can be placed on grill for further authentic taste.

CAULIFLOWER & CHIVE MASH WITH/ SWEET CARROTS

- 1 pound cauliflower
- ¼ cup fresh chopped chives
- pinch mashed garlic
- ½ pound small baby carrots
- ½ tsp chopped fresh parsley
- ½ cup fresh pineapple
- fresh mint leaves

Marinate carrots in pineapple juice add chop parsleys right before serving garnish with fresh mint in a food processor pure' cauliflower and garlic

Fold into a serving bowl and fold in chopped chives

CASSAVA WITH SPICY SOFRITO

- Cassava
- Cilantro
- 2 cup chopped seeded tomato
- 1 cup chopped onion
- 1 cup chopped green pepper
- 2 scotch bonnet
- olive oil
- veggie broth
- add salt if desired
- 4 clove garlic

In a blender or food processor put 2 bunch cilantro,onions,peppers scotch bonnet and garlic add olive oil cut and peel cassava in rounds 2 inch wide cook cassava in veggie broth till tender add sofrito and simmer down good with rice.

COCO RICE

- 2 cups rice
- ½ cup coconut milk
- ¼ cup shredded coconut
- 3-4 whole scallions

Cook rice in coconut milk and water bring to boil cut roots off scallion and fold in rice lower and simmer till rice is done toast shredded coconut spoon rice in serving bowl and top with toasted coconut.

CURRY AND PINEAPPLE FRIED RICE

- 1medium onion (chopped)
- 4 carrots (julienne)
- ¼ lb snow peas (trimmed)
- 2 to 5 T vegetable oil
- 1 to 2 T curry powder
- 2 T cilantro (chopped)
- 1 T lemon juice
- 2 cups pineapple chunks
- 1 cup baby corn
- 4 cups cooked white or brown rice

In a pot of boiling water, partially cook the onions, carrots and snow peas for about 3 minutes. Plunge the vegetables into cold water, drain and set aside. In a large skillet, heat the oil. Stir in the curry and pineapple, cook stirring for 1 minute. Add the rice and stir fry for 5 minutes more. Stir in baby corn, lemon juice, cilantro and cooked vegetables. Cook until hot.

REGGAE RICE

- 2 cups of hot cooked rice
- 2 tablespoon of mango chutney
- 1/4 teaspoon of ground ginger
- 1/2 cup of chopped red pepper
- 1/3 cup of sliced green onions
- 1/2 cup of slivered almonds, toasted
- 11 ounce canned mandarin oranges, drained
- 8 ounces canned crushed pineapple, drained
- 1/1 cup of unsweetened grated coconut, toasted

In a large size skillet combine rice, mandarin oranges, pineapple, red pepper, almonds, green onions, coconut, chutney along with the ginger over medium high heat. Now stir and cook it until the ingredients are well blended and thoroughly heated. To toast the coconut, spread grated coconut on an ungreased baking sheet then toast at 300 F. for 1 minute.

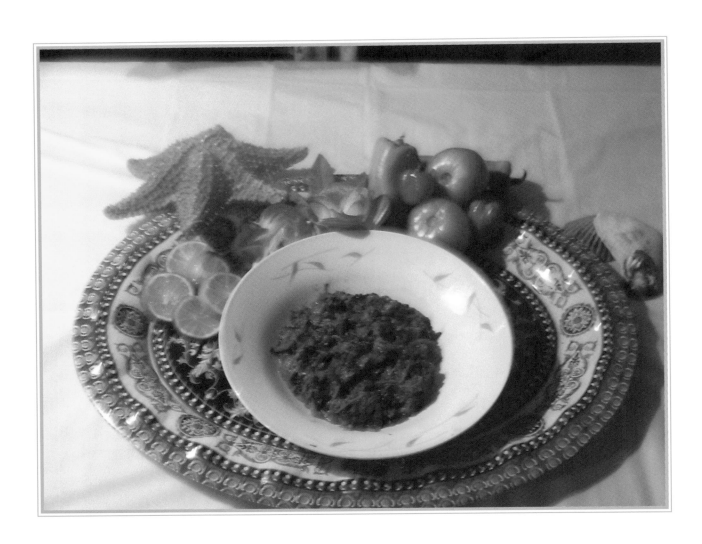

DO YOU CALLOU

- 1 pound callou
- ½ cup chopped onion
- ½ cup chopped green bell pepper
- ¼ cup chopped seeded tomato
- 1 half scotch bonnet chopped
- 1T smoked soy chips
- olive oil
- 1 tsp lime juice

Sauté onions, peppers, garlic and scotch bonnet in olive oil, fold in callou and tomato add veggie broth and simmer till callou is tender.

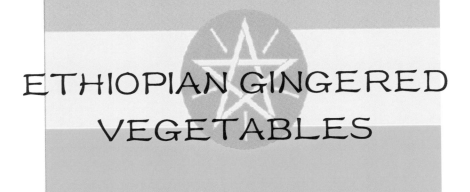

ETHIOPIAN GINGERED VEGETABLES

- green chilies, skinned, seeded and chopped
- teaspoon fresh ginger, grated
- small potatoes, cubed
- 1/2 lb green beans
- carrots, cut in strips
- water, as needed
- medium onions, quartered and separated
- tablespoons olive oil
- garlic cloves
- salt and pepper, to taste if desired

Place potatoes, green beans, and carrots into boiling salted water, cover, and cook 5 minutes remove veggies and rinse.

Sauté the Chile and onion in oil until soft but not brown.

Add the ginger, garlic, salt, and pepper and sauté 5 minutes

Add the rest of ingredients, stir well, and cook over medium heat until veggies are tender

ETHIOPIAN GREEN PEAS

- 1 bag dried whole green peas
- ½ cup onion (chopped)
- ½ cup green bell pepper (chopped)
- 4 cloves garlic (mashed)
- 1 T lemon juice
- 1 T paprika
- 1 tsp coriander
- ½ tsp ground ginger
- 4 cups water
- salt if desired

In a large bowl soak peas over night. Drain peas and add to a large pot with water. Then add all remaining ingredients. Bring to a boil. Then cook until just tender. Serve with Injera.

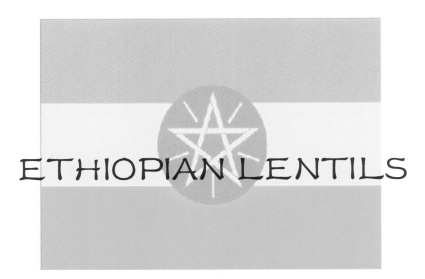

ETHIOPIAN LENTILS

- 1lb lentils
- 1 bell pepper (chopped) + 1 14oz green chilies
- 6 cups mild green chilies (roasted, peeled and seeded)
- 2 red onions (chopped)
- 2 or more cloves garlic (minced)
- 2 T BereBere seasoning
- freshly ground black pepper
- 6 cups water or vegetable broth

Bring lentils and broth or water to a boil and simmer for 10 minutes. Add chilies, onion, peppers, garlic and BereBere mix. Cook covered for another 30 minutes. Until most liquid is absorbed. Serve with Brown rice

And sliced tomatoes. Fresh ground pepper to taste.

FRIED BROWN RICE

- 2 cups cooked brown rice
- ½ cup onion (chopped)
- ½ cup scallions (chopped)
- 1 cup cooked sweet green peas
- ½ cup carrot (chopped)
- 1 T soy sauce
- olive oil
- ¼ cup vegetable stock (for deglazing)
- red pepper flakes if desired

In a large sauté pan with olive oil sauté onions and scallions first. Then add in peas, carrots and rice. Sauté for about 5 minutes more. Then deglaze the rice mixture with the vegetable broth and soy sauce. Sprinkle with red pepper flakes if desired.

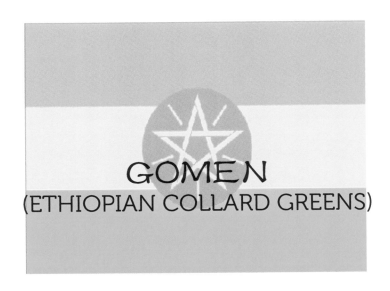

GOMEN
(ETHIOPIAN COLLARD GREENS)

- 1 bunch collard greens
- 1 medium onion, chopped (optional)
- 1 tablespoon niter kebbeh (Ethiopian butter)
- salt and pepper to taste

Wash the greens well and drain.

Cut and remove the coarse part off of the ends of the stems.

Chop the leaves coarsely and set aside. In a pot, heat up some niter kebbeh. Add the onion, and some salt. Sauté until the onion turns clear and has softened. Add the collard leaves and stir well. Cook until tender adding a small amount of water if necessary to help the greens steam. Season with salt and pepper and arrange on injera with some other stews.

HAITIAN RICE & BEANS

- ½ dry kidney beans
- 4 tablespoons olive oil
- 1 bulb shallot, minced
- 3 cloves garlic, minced
- 2 cup long grain white rice
- 2 bay leaves
- 1 tablespoon kosher salt
- freshly ground black pepper to taste
- 1/4 teaspoon ground cloves
- 3 sprigs fresh parsley
- 3 sprigs fresh thyme
- 1 scotch bonnet pepper
- 4 cups water (for rice) 2 ½ cups water (for beans)

Place beans in a large pot, cover with 2 ½ cups water. Bring to a boil, reduce heat, and simmer 1 1/2 hours, or until tender. Drain, reserving liquid. Heat oil in a large skillet over medium heat. Sauté shallot and garlic until fragrant. Stir in cooked beans, and cook for 2 minutes. Measure reserved liquid, and add water to equal 4 cups; stir into skillet. Stir in the uncooked rice. Season with bayleaves, salt, pepper, and cloves. Place sprigs of parsley and thyme, and scotch bonnet pepper on top, and bring to a boil. Reduce heat, cover, and simmer for 18 to 20 minutes. Remove bay leaves to serve.

JERK VEGGIE STIR FRY

- 1 bunch broccoli (stemmed)
- 1 cup carrots (julienne)
- 1 cup yellow bell pepper (sliced thin)
- 1 cup red bell pepper (sliced thin)
- 1 cup green bell pepper (sliced thin)
- 1 cup onion (sliced thin)
- ½ cup jimica (julienne)
- ¼ cup pineapple chunks
- 2 T jerk seasoning
- 1 tsp ground ginger
- peanut oil for frying

In a skillet sauté onions, peppers, jimica and carrots in peanut oil. Cook for 5 minutes then add broccoli, pineapple chinks and ground ginger. Cook for 3 more minutes. Then add jerk seasoning and stir well for 5 minutes. Serve with rice.

JOLL OF RICE

- 1 cup dry black eye peas
- 2 large onions (chopped)
- 2 cloves garlic (minced)
- 1 green bell pepper (chopped)
- 1 lb carrots (chopped)
- 2 jalapenos pepper (seeded & chopped)
- 3 T ground ginger
- 1 stalk celery (chopped)
- 4 large tomatoes (seeded & chopped)
- ½ lb green beans
- 1 ½ T tomato paste
- 2 tsp cayenne pepper
- 2 tsp curry powder
- 1 package sazon
- 1 ½ T canola oil
- 1 ½ cups uncooked brown rice
- 3 quarts vegetable stock or water

In a large bowl soak peas overnight in 1 quart of water, drain. Add 2 quarts vegetable stock or water to the peas in a large pot, and simmer for 15 minutes. Drain and set aside the cooked vegetable stock or water. Heat oil in a Dutch oven or casserole dish. Add onion, 1 T ground ginger, 1 jalapeno pepper, 1 clove garlic and bell pepper. Cook stirring for 5 minutes. Add remaining onion, ginger, jalapeno, garlic, cooked vegetable stock or water, tomatoes, tomato paste, cayenne, curry powder and sazon. Simmer for 10 minutes. Add peas, carrots and rice. Cook for 5 minutes more. Then add green beans. Simmer for 15 minutes. Preheat oven to 400 degrees. Cover the casserole dish bake for 30 minutes.

POTATO CURRIED

- 4 tsp curry powder
- 1 small onion, cut into small pieces
- 4 cloves garlic, minced or crushed
- 2 medium sized potatoes

Use sharp knife to slice potatoes in wedges.

Use a large pan to heat the spices in the oil on medium heat but do not burn. Add onion and garlic and cook 2 minutes.

Cook potatoes for 2 additional minutes. Add the water and cook potatoes until tender on medium heat.

PRINCESS KAYA'S OKRA & STEWED TOMATOES

- 1 cup onion (coarsely chopped)
- 1 cup green bell pepper (coarsely chopped)
- 4 cloves garlic (minced)
- 1 stalk celery (coarsely chopped)
- 1 lb cherry tomatoes halved
- 1 lb okra fresh (frozen optional)
- 1 package sazon
- ¼ cup water
- 3 T olive oil
- ¼ cup chopped parsley
- 1 pinch coriander
- fresh ground black pepper to taste

Sautee onions, bell pepper, garlic, and celery in olive oil. Add in sazon, coriander, and parsley. Then stir in halved tomatoes. Stir for about 3 minutes. Add in okra and water. Simmer for 30 minutes. Serve with brown rice and flat bread.

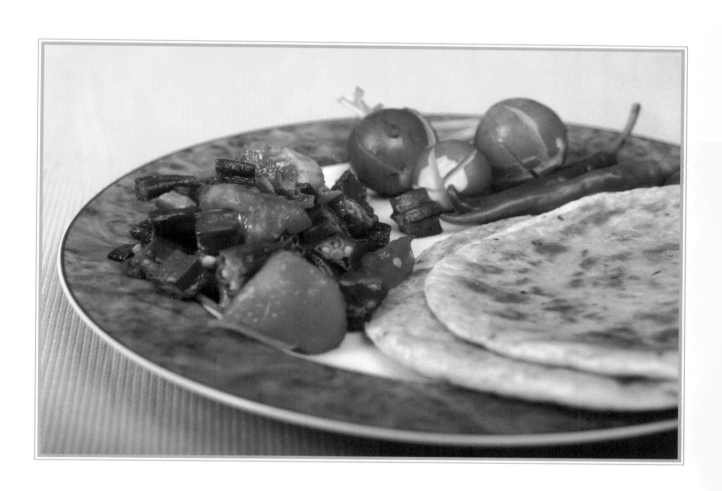

SEARED SEASAME TOFU

- 1 pound tofu
- ½ cup sesame oil
- 2 T sesame seeds
- 1 T garlic powder
- orange juice
- olive oil
- soy sauce

Marinate tofu in sesame oil, orange juice and garlic powder overnight in fridge. Pan Sear in sesame oil add more if not enough from marinate add little more orange juice and the soy sauce to deglaze top with sesame seeds and slice to serve.

STUFFED CABBAGE

- 1 whole Savoy cabbage
- 1 cup cooked wild rice
- ½ cup chopped onion
- ½ cup chopped yellow bell pepper
- 1tsp dried sage
- ½ cup tomatoes sauce
- 1 whole seeded chopped tomatoes

Pull leaves off cabbage whole cook till softened slightly cook wild rice with onions, peppers and tomato add sage stuff rice mixture in whole leave and roll place in baking dish in rows close together spread tomatoes sauce over top bake 30 minutes or till browned slightly and bubbling.

STUFFED YELLOW PEPPER

- 4-6 yellow peppers
- ¼ cup mango (chopped)
- ¼ cup onion (chopped)
- ¼ cup green bell pepper
- ¼ cup tomatoes (seeded & chopped)
- ½ tsp garlic powder
- ½ tsp dried thyme
- 1 jalapeno pepper (seeded & chopped) (optional)
- 2 cups brown rice (cooked)
- 4 cups vegetable stock (for brown rice)
- olive oil

Preheat oven to 350

Precook 2 cups brown rice in 4 cups vegetable stock. Set aside. In a skillet sauté onions, bell peppers and jalapeno (optional). Then add in tomatoes, mangos, garlic powder and thyme. Cook for about 5 minutes. Then add in brown rice. Stir together and set aside. Cut the tops off each pepper (set aside), and carefully scoop out seeds and membrane. Spoon in the rice mixture. Filling up each pepper. Place the tops back on each pepper. Place the peppers in a square or rectangle baking dish. Bake for 25 minutes.

SWEET & HOT VEGGIE STIR

- 1pound long green bean
- ½ pound snow peas
- 1 cup thin sliced red bell pepper
- 1 cup thin sliced red onion
- 1T sesame seeds
- 1 cup juice from orange
- 1 cup juice from lime
- ½ cup juice from lemon
- 1 cup sliced pineapple
- pinch scotch bonnet pepper
- ½ tsp grated or mashed garlic

In a small bowl whisk together the citrus juice from orange, lime and lemon add in grated garlic and hot pepper till all is blended. After you have washed and trim, and slice veggies and pineapple mix in a large bowl toss together with citrus dressing.

TOMATO & LENTIL COUCOUS

- Couscous
- 1 cup chopped seeded tomato
- ¼ cup chopped onion
- 1 cup cooked red lentil
- 2 cups veggie broth

Follow directions on back couscous, using veggie broth. Bring to boil and simmer. Fold in tomato, lentil and onion. Simmer for about 20 minutes more. Let it stand for 5-10 minutes.

TOMATO CASSOROLE

- 1 medium potato, peeled and cut into 1/2-inch pieces
- 1 medium yam, peeled and cut into 1/2-inch pieces
- 1 red bell pepper, seeded and cut into 1/2-inch pieces
- 2 carrots, peeled and cut into 1/2-inch pieces
- 5 tablespoons olive oil
- 1 red onion, thinly sliced into rings
- 2 small or 1 large zucchini, cut crosswise into 1/4-inch-thick pieces pepper
- 2 large ripe tomatoes, cut crosswise into 1/4-inch thick slices
- 1/2 cup grated Parmesan
- 2 tablespoons dried wheat bread crumbs
- Fresh basil sprigs, for garnish
- Fresh sprigs lemon thyme

Preheat the oven to 400 degrees F.

Toss the potato, yam, bell pepper, carrots, and 2 tablespoons of olive oil in a 13 by 9 by 2-inch baking dish to coat. Sprinkle with pepper and toss until coated. Spread vegetables evenly over the bottom of the pan.

Arrange the onion slices evenly over the vegetable mixture. Arrange the zucchini over the onion. Drizzle with 2 tablespoons of oil. Sprinkle with pepper. Arrange the tomato slices over the zucchini. Stir the Parmesan and bread crumbs in a small bowl to blend. Sprinkle the Parmesan bread crumbs over the vegetables in the baking dish. Drizzle with the last tablespoon of olive oil. Bake uncovered until the vegetables are tender, and the topping is golden brown, about 40 minutes. Garnish with fresh basil sprigs, if desired

YAM HASH

- 2-3 sweet potato
- 2-3 yellow yams
- ¼ cup chopped onions
- 1 T parsley
- 2 T wheat flour
- oil for frying

Peel and cut yams and potato dust with wheat flour in small cube size dust with wheat flour brown in oil add in onions brown till tender and golden brown sprinkle with parsley.

VEGETABLE ALECHA

The Copts in Ethiopia have many fast days on which they are not permitted to eat meat. Vegetables Alechas and Wats are substituted on these days. (The Wat differs from the Alecha in that it is made with a spice called Ber-beri or Awaze.)

In a 4-quart saucepan:
- Sauté 1 cup Bermuda onions
- Add 4 potatoes cut in thick slices
- 4 T oil until soft but not brown.
- Add 4 carrots, peeled and cut in 1-inch slices
- 4 green peppers, cleaned and cut in quarters
- 3 cups water
- 1 6-oz. can tomato sauce
- 2 tsp salt
- 1/2 tsp ground ginger

Cook for 10 minutes covered. Plunge 2 tomatoes in boiling water, remove skins, cut in 8 wedges each, and add to stew. Cover and cook for 10 minutes Add 8 cabbage wedges, 1 inch wide. Cook until vegetables are tender Cook until vegetables are tender.

WARM BREEZE SPEGHETTI

- 1 pound wheat spaghetti
- ½ cup chopped onion
- ½ cup chopped green bell pepper
- 2 cup cut tomato
- 2 cup fresh callou
- 1 tsp dried thyme
- ¼ cup fresh basil
- 1 tsp dried oregano
- 1 T garlic powder
- 1 whole clove garlic mashed and chopped
- olive oil

Cook wheat spaghetti till tender don't over cook, cut tomatoes in cubed bite size peaces not to small. sauté garlic onions and peppers in olive oil till just light translucent add tomatoes and callou and cook till slightly tender don't over cook to avoid mushy veggies fold in to wheat spaghetti add fresh basil at the end will have more flavor serve warm.

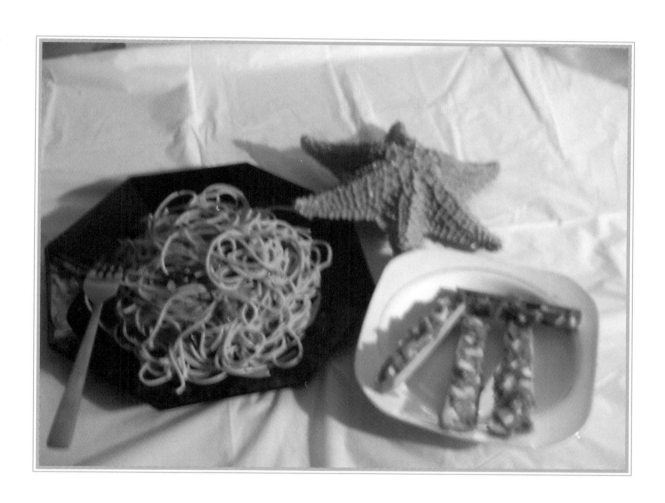

SALADS AND DRESSINGS

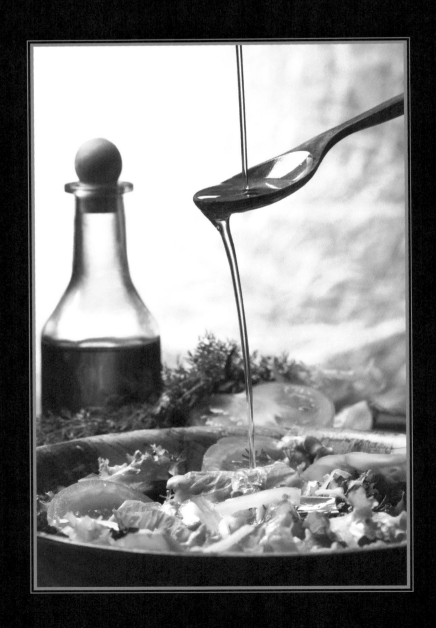

BAHAMIAN COLE SLAW

- 1 bag prewashed and cut Cole slaw mix
- ½ cup red onion (finely chopped)
- ¼ cup pineapple juice
- 1 cup soy mayonnaise
- ¼ cup vinegar
- 1 whole seeded jalapeno pepper (chopped)
- ½ cup pineapple (chopped)

In a large bowl combine all ingredients. Let chill for 30 minutes or more.

BLACK OLIVE DRESSING

- ¼ cup Balsamic Vinegar
- 2/3cup extra virgin olive oil
- 2 T dijion mustard
- 1 T honey
- ½ cup chopped pitted black olives
- 1 T oregano

Wisk together vinegar, olive oil, honey and mustard. Add in olives and oregano last serve over favorite salad

BROCCO SLAW

- 1 bunch broccoli
- ½ cup chopped red onion
- 1 cup chopped seeded tomato
- ½ cup shredded carrots
- ½ cup veggie or soy mayo
- ½ tsp raw sugar
- 1 T red wine vinegar
- ½ cup shredded veggie cheeses for garnish

Wash broccoli and dry cut off tops the florets and cut in half once add chopped red onion and carrots whish mayo and vinegar add sugar fold into salad garnish with shredded veggie cheeses

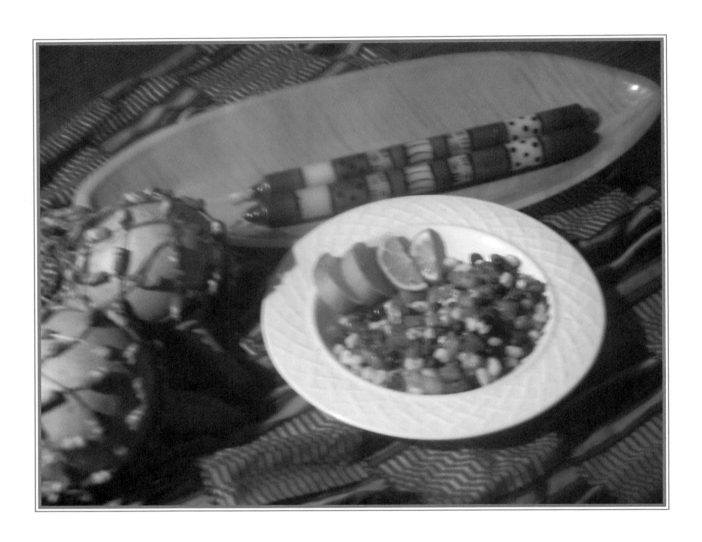

CARNIVAL SALAD

- 3 cups cooked corn
- 2cup cooked black beans
- 2cup cooked red beans
- 2 cup seeded chopped tomato
- ¼ cup chopped roasted red bell pepper
- ¼ cup chopped red onion
- ½ chopped jalapeño pepper seeded
- ¼ cup olive oil
- ½ cup red wine vinegar
- 1 tsp paprika
- 1 T garlic powder
- 2T chopped cilantro
- pinch saffron

Mix all beans and corn in bowl chop peppers and onions and add seasonings whisk herbs in with olive oil and vinegar pour over salad and chill at least ½ hour

CHICK PEA & AVOCADO SALAD WITH LEMON DRESSING

- 3 cups fresh spinach
- 3 cups romaine lettuce
- 3 cups iceberg lettuce (shredded thin)
- 1 cup arugula
- 1 cup chickpea
- ½ cup thin sliced red onion
- whole avocado sliced
- 1T chives
- 1 T parsley

DRESSING; 1 T lemon zest 2/3 cup extra virgin olive oil and1/2 cup red wine vinegar Whisk till blended add chives and parsley

Rinse drain and dry lettuces, arugula and spinach. Toss in bowl with chickpeas and red onions make dressing and fold in to salad place sliced avocado slices on top of salad

EGYPTIAN POTATO SALAD

- 1 pound potato
- ½ cup chopped red onion
- ½ cup chopped green bell pepper
- 1 cup cooked green peas
- ¼ cup extra virgin olive oil
- ½ cup shredded carrots
- ½ tsp coriander

Peel and cook potato till fork tender cut potato in cubes fold in chopped veggies and add seasonings toss with olive oil

Add salt to taste and ground black pepper

EMPRESS SALAD

- 1 pint cherry tomato
- 1 pint yellow cherry tomato
- 1 cup thin sliced red onion
- 1 cup sliced thin seedless cucumber
- ¼ cup chopped fine green bell pepper
- ½ tsp lemon thyme
- 1 tsp chopped cilantro
- ¼ cup vinegar
- 1 T lemon juice
- ¼ cup extra virgin olive oil
- 1-2 bunch romaine lettuce

Cut cherry tomatoes in half once

Mix tomatoes and chopped peppers together fold in cucumber slices and onions (cucumber and onions should be sliced in half thin slices add thyme and basil mix together well on a serving plate lay romaine lettuce down and place tomato salad in center of lettuce.

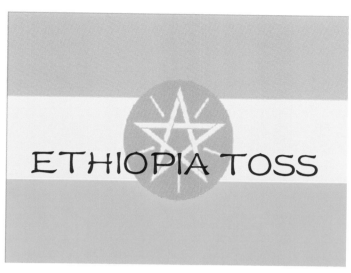

ETHIOPIA TOSS

- 1 whole lettuce
- 2 cups sliced cucumber
- 1 cup sliced red onion
- 2 cups sliced and seeded tomato
- 2-3 cooked boil egg

This salad is in layers

Use large serving plate making layers starting with lettuce next layer cucumber top with sliced tomato place sliced thin red onion top layer is sliced boiled egg serve with Injera or flat bread

MY FATHER'S BREAKFAST SALAD #1

- 4 cups shredded carrots
- 1 cup raisins (or chopped grapes)
- ¼ cup soy mayo
- ½ tsp raw sugar
- ½ cup chopped papaya

After shredding the carrots (should be about 6-8 carrots) [1]mix in bowl with fruit whisk mayo and raw sugar and add to salad chill and serve

MY FATHER'S SUPPER SALAD

- 1 pound cooked pasta
- 1 cup chopped tomato
- ½ cup chopped fine onion
- ½ cup soy mayo
- ¼ cup shredded carrots
- 1 T parsley

After pasta is tender rinse with cool water and drain add chopped onions, tomatoes, carrots and mayo salt and pepper to taste let chill

FREEDOM FRUIT SALAD

- 2 cup sliced bananas
- 1 cup papaya
- 1 cup mango
- 1 cup chopped pineapple
- 2 cup mandarin orange
- 1 whole star fruit sliced
- 1 cup melon
- 1 whole orange
- 1 whole lemon
- 1 whole lime
- 1 cup toasted shredded coconut
- 1/2 cup chopped mint

Peel and slice fruit, cut in chunks or bite size pieces. In a bowl toss fruit and squeeze the juice from the orange, lemon and the lime it will prevent fruit from turning brown. Toast coconut till lightly browned add into fruit mixture toss in chopped mint and place sliced star fruit on top

KINGS RICE SALAD

- 1 cup wild rice
- ½ cup brown rice
- ½ cup seeded chopped tomato
- 1 tsp dried thyme
- 1 T parsley
- ½ dried sage
- ½ tsp paprika
- ½ tsp garlic powder
- ¼ cup extra virgin olive oil
- ¼ cup red wine vinegar

Cook rice and let cool completely loosen with fork so will cool fluffier and able to separate easy. After rice is cool fold and loosen more with fork in salad bowl and add remaining ingrdeances whisk olive oil and vinegar and fold in rice salad chill before serving.

MANDARIN ORANGE VINEGARETTE

- ¼ cup mandarin oranges
- 1 T dried thyme
- 1T lemon juice
- ½ cup white wine vinegar
- ¼ cup olive oil

In bowl whisk vinegar lemon juice and thyme whisk in oil fold in oranges serve over veggies or salad

ORANGE TOSSED UP

- 1 cup orange segments
- 2cup fresh spinach
- 1 cup sliced thin red onion
- ½ cup sunflower seed
- ½ cup alfalfa sprouts
- ½ cup sliced thin yellow bell pepper
- ½ cup chopped broccoli florets

Salad dressing of your choice

We suggest our mandarin orange dressing

PINEAPPLE DRESSING

- 1 cup olive oil
- ½ cup pineapple juice
- 3 T lime juice
- ½ T sugar
- 3 T apple cider vinegar
- 3 T fresh cilantro (chopped)
- 1/2 T kosher salt (optional)

In a bowl whish together pineapple juice, lime juice, sugar, vinegar, salt and cilantro. Then slowly whisk in olive oil. Serve with your favorite salad.

RASTA PASTA

- 1 pound Tri color pasta
- ¼ cup chopped red onion
- ¼ cup chopped green bell pepper
- ¼ cup chopped red bell pepper
- ¼ cup chopped yellow bell pepper
- 1 T copped fresh basil
- 1 T dried thyme
- ½ cup steamed zucchini
- ½ cup steamed yellow squash (or yellow pumpkin)
- 1 clove chopped mashed garlic
- ¼ cup favorite dressings (see dressings)
- 10 to 12 green figs

Cook pasta till ala dente (slightly tender) steam zucchini and yellow squash with mashed garlic fold in to pasta with remaining ingrdeances add dressing and chill salad

ROASTED PEPPER MAYO

- ¼ cup roasted red bell pepper
- 8 oz soybean mayo
- 1tsp oregano
- 1tsp basil
- 1 tsp thyme

In a blender or processor blend mayo, peppers and seasonings keep cool serve on salads veggies or sandwiches

ROOTS BREAD SALAD

- 1 Whole loaf french bread
- 1 Whole loaf itailian bread
- 1 Whole loaf wheat bread
- 1 Red oion cut in slithers
- 1 Cup cherry tomatoes cut in half once
- 1 Cup yellow cherry tomatoes cut in half once
- 1 Cup red wine vinegar
- ¼ Cup extra virgian olive oil
- 1 T lemon juice
- 1 T garlic powder
- 1 T dried basil
- 1 T dried parsely

Lightly toast bread till just slightly toast cut in squares. Set aside in a large bowl.

In another small bowl mix vinegar, olive oil, lemon juice, garlic, basil, and parsley.

Mix well add in tomatoes, and red onions. Toss dressing mix to bread when serving.

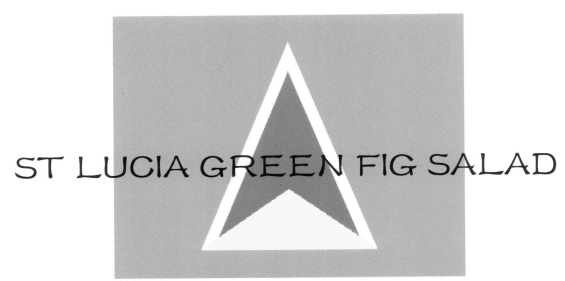

ST LUCIA GREEN FIG SALAD

- 1 egg
- 1 lime
- 1 onion
- mayonnaise
- 1 cup of oil
- 2 sweet peppers
- 6 green bananas
- salt and pepper

First boil, and peel the green figs.

Allow to cool, then dice and place in a bowl.

Next add the prepared onions, sweet peppers, and the boiled egg, now add the mayonnaise.

SWEET & SPICY LEMON DRESSING

- ¼ cup lemon juice
- ¼ tsp lemon zest
- 1 ½ tsp honey
- ¼ tsp ground cumin
- ¼ tsp ground cinnamon
- ¼ tsp ground ginger
- ½ tsp cayenne pepper
- ¼ cup extra-virgin olive oil
- Freshly ground pepper to taste

Whisk all ingredients together, slowly adding the olive oil. Serve over your favorite salad.

WARM CLYPSO SALAD

- 1 cup chopped mango
- 1 cup cooked red bean
- ½ cup cooked black beans
- ¼ cup chopped celery
- ¼ cup chopped onion
- ¼ cup seeded chopped tomato
- 1 T chopped fresh cilantro
- 1 T thyme
- ½ lime juiced
- ½ orange juiced
- ½ chopped scotch bonnet

While beans are still warm and drained, add chopped mango, tomatoes and the rest of the ingredients together squeeze 1 half lime and 1 half orange and toss, serve warm over lettuce

SWEETS

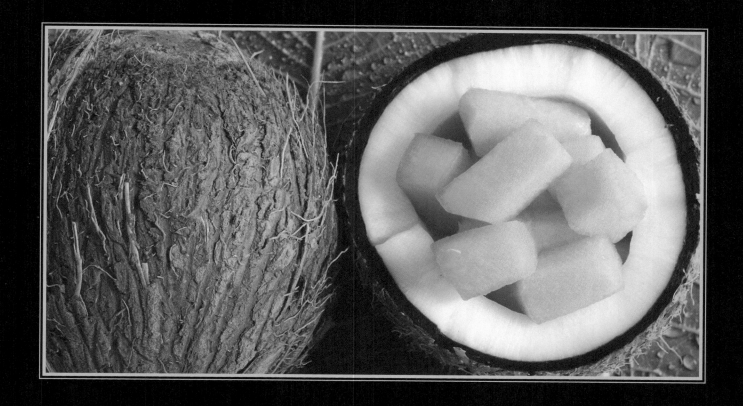

AFRICAN COCONUT ALMOND CONGO BARS

- 2 cups flaked coconut
- 1 tsp baking powder
- 2 cups all-purpose flour
- 1 cup soy butter, softened at room temperature
- 1 ½ cups light brown sugar, firmly packed
- 2 eggs, lightly beaten
- 1 tsp vanilla extract
- 1 tsp almond extract
- 1 cup almond slivers

All ingredients should be allowed to come to room temperature if they have been in the refrigerator. Preheat oven to 350° F.

Mix together the baking powder, and flour.

When oven is hot, place the coconut on a cookie sheet and toast until lightly browned (one or two minutes). Remove and let cool.

Using an electric mixer, mix together the butter and brown sugar. Add the beaten egg 1 by 1 mixing well. Add vanilla and almond extract. Stir in the flour mixture. Mix well then gently stir in alomonds and cocnut.

Lightly grease (or butter) and flour a 9- x 13-inch cake pan. Spread the batter into the pan. Bake at 350° F for about 25 minutes.

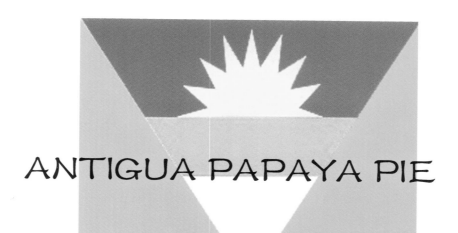

ANTIGUA PAPAYA PIE

- 4 egg Whites
- -a pinch of cinnamon
- 4 tablespoons of flour
- 4 tablespoons of sugar
- 3 Ripe medium papayas
- 2 teaspoons of lime juice
- 1/2 teaspoon of lime zest
- 1 dash of orange extract
- 1 Sweet Medium Pre baked
- -pie Shell

Remove the seeds and coarsely mash the papayas. Now add the lime juice, zest, cinnamon and the orange extract. Fold in the sugar and flour.

Now beat the egg whites together until they are stiff then fold into mixture.

Finally, bake for at least twenty five minutes until the top are brown. Serve warm or cold

CARIBBEAN BANANA DESSERT

- 1 cup of soy milk
- 1 cup of breadcrumbs
- 1/3 cup of brown sugar
- 3 cups of banana chunks
- 1 tablespoon of lemon zest
- 1 tablespoon of orange zest
- 1 tablespoon of lemon juice
- 3 tablespoons of orange juice
- -mixed with 4 tablespoons of Water
- 3 tablespoons of pineapple juice
- 2 tablespoons of soy margarine, melted and cooled

Preheat oven to 300 F. Oil a 1 1/2 quart mould.

Combine peels & juices with banana & set aside.

Place egg replacer, sugar & pineapple juice in a food processor & pulse till blended.

Add soy milk & bread crumbs & pulse a few more times. Spoon mixture over banana mixture. Next add the margarine then mix well and pour right into prepared mold.

Place the mould into a large size pan then pour in enough of the boiling water to reach 1/2 way up the sides of mould. Bake for about 1 hour 20 minutes, a knife inserted should come out clean.

Finally you may have to add more boiling water during the cooking time. Cool off for 20 to 30 minutes and remove from the mould. Refrigerate 2 hours before serving.

CARROT BREAD

- 2 eggs
- 1/2 cup of flour
- 1 cups of walnuts
- 1/4 cups of raw sugar
- 1 cup of salad oil
- 1 teaspoon of vanilla
- 1/2. teaspoon of salt
- 1 1/2 teaspoon of cinnamon
- 1 1/2 cup of carrot pieces
- 1 1/2 teaspoon of baking soda

Heat the oven to 350 F. and grease 9" x 5" loaf pan. Sift together the flour, baking soda, salt and cinnamon into large mixing bowl. Set aside.

Chop the nuts into blender or with sharp knife.

Add to dry ingredients. 4. Mix sugar, eggs, off and vanilla until smooth in blender.

Add the carrot pieces to mixture in blender and liquefy. Pour over dry ingredients and mix only until dry ingredients are moistened. Pour in a pan and bake for 1 hr. or until tester comes out clean. Cool for 5 minutes.

COCONUT CANDY

- 2 cups grated coconut
- 1 1/2 cups of sugar
- 1/2 cup of water
- 2 tsp vanilla extract
- 1 tsp cinnamon powder
- 1/4 tsp baking powder

Bring water to a boil and add coconut

Cook for 5- 10 minutes and add sugar.

Sit constantly and cook for additional 25 minutes until coconut hardens.

Remove from heat and add remaining ingredients.

Place spoonfuls on a plate or wax sheet and allow cooling and hardening.

COCONUT SHILINGS

- Buckwheat pancake mix
- ½ cup coconut
- butter
- ½ tsp vanilla extract

In bowl mix pancake mixture with water, add in coconut and vanilla extract. Butter a skillet or pan. With a ladle pour batter to make small pancakes. Brown on both sides. Serve with favorite syrup

FRESH COCONUT POT DU CRÈME

- 1 quart heavy cream
- 1 vanilla bean, split in half
- 1 cup coco cream
- 2 cups fresh coconut
- 10 egg yolks

Preheat oven to 300 degrees F. Combine the cream, scraped vanilla, whole vanilla bean, and coconut milk in a sauce pan over medium heat. Bring the cream up to a boil and reduce to a simmer. Simmer the cream for 5 minutes. Remove from the heat and discard the vanilla bean. In an electric mixer, beat the yolks. Gradually pour the hot cream into the mixer. Mix until incorporated. Strain the liquid into a pitcher. Fold in the fresh coconut. Place eight (3/4 cup) ramekins in a roasting pan. Fill the ramekins to the rim with the custard. Pour water into the roasting pan 1/2 way up the sides of the ramekins. Cover the pan loosely with foil and bake for 1 to 1 1/2 hours or until set. Remove from the pan and let the custards cool completely. Place in the refrigerator and chill for 1 hour. Garnish with whipped cream, chocolate shavings.

GRAPE FRUIT GRINATA

- 10 oz grapefruit juice
- 4 oz orange juice

In a freezer safe bowl freeze juices for about 15 minutes. Scrape mixture with a fork. Continue the process until mixture forms into water ice.

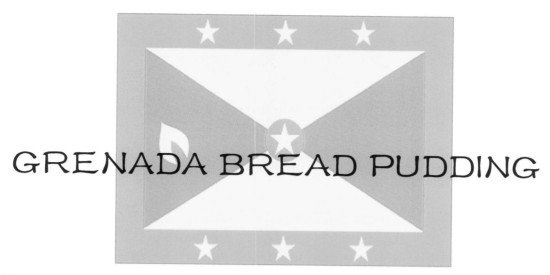

GRENADA BREAD PUDDING

- 3 large eggs
- 2 cups of milk
- 1/2 cup of raisins
- 5 cups of cubed bread
- 1 1/2 teaspoons of vanilla extract
- 1 1/4 teaspoons of nutmeg (ground)
- 6 ounces Morne Delice Nutmeg Syrup

First in a large bowl mix together all the ingredients except for the

Bread cubes, raisins, place the bread cubes on a greased loaf pan. Fold in egg mixture with the raisins.

Let it stand for about 45 minutes, patting bread down into the liquid occasionally.

Next place into a preheated 350 F.

Oven and bake for at least 40 minutes.

I-N- I LOVE TARTS

- 10-12 puff pastry cups (frozen section)
- 1 cup berries
- orange juice
- 1 T ground ginger
- 1 T ground nutmeg
- 1 T cornstarch
- pineapple juice

In sauce pan warm berries in juices and spices add corn starch till fruit thicken bake pastry cups till golden brown fold in fruit mixture serve with dolce' or crème fresh

ITAL PIE

- 2 cup sun dried guava paste
- 1 cup grounded fine nuts (can soak)
- 1 cup shredded coconut
- 2 cup sliced thin banana
- sliced thin mango
- sliced thin papaya
- sliced thin melon of choice
- sliced thin star fruit (for garnish)
- orange, lemon, lime

Soak fruit with juice to prevent browning, drain fruit. Mix ground nuts, coconut and 1 cup guava paste together till forms thick ball press into pie dish to form shell. Place sliced fruit in layers in between layers of fruit. Spread guava paste. Press fruit firmly. Fill to top of pie shell let sit several hours in direct sun is best slice pie and serve.

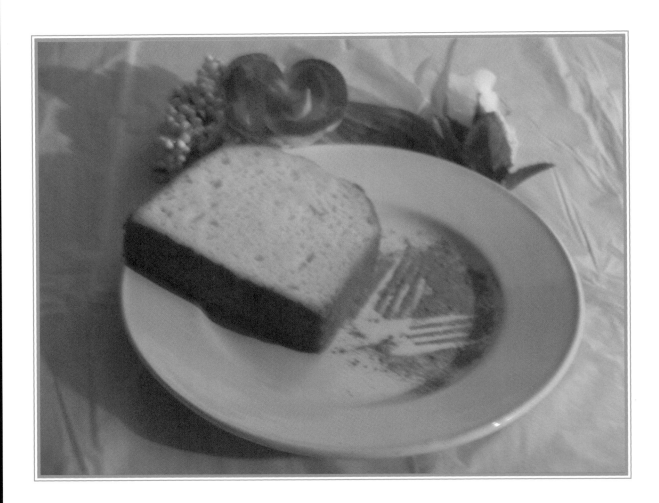

NANA'S 7UP CAKE

- 3 cups flour
- 3 cups sugar
- 2 ½ sticks butter
- 5 eggs
- ½ tsp salt
- 1 tsp vanilla extract
- 8 oz 7 up or cherry 7 up

Preheat oven to 350. Greased a bunt or deep round cake pan.

In a mixer mix sugar, salt, vanilla and butter, then slowly add in flour. (Remember to scrape sides of bowl to insure all is mixed well) Add in 7 up, then one by one add in eggs. Until mixed well. Pour batter in baking pan. Bake for 35 minutes or poke with a toothpick to test if it comes out clean. Then let cool.

We make it for special occasions.

PRINCE AMIR TROPICAL COLADA CAKE

- 2 pounds of fresh pineapple, peeled, cored and cubed
- 2 1/2 cups sugar
- 1 teaspoon ground cinnamon, in all
- 1 teaspoon grated nutmeg, in all
- 1 ½ cup coconut
- 1/2 sticks butter, softened, in all
- 1 teaspoon baking powder
- 1 teaspoon baking soda
- 2 whole eggs
- 1 teaspoon vanilla
- 1 cup milk
- 2 1/4 cups flour
- 1/2 teaspoon nutmeg
- 1/2 teaspoon cinnamon

Preheat oven 350 degrees F. In a mixing bowl, toss the pineapple with coconut and 1 cup of brown sugar, 1/2 teaspoon cinnamon, and 1/2 teaspoon nutmeg. Place pineapple and coconut in a greased cake pan pour cake batter over and bake 1hour.

PRINCEES NYKEMAH ORANGE COLADA CAKE

- 2 cup mandarin oranges
- 1 ½ cup coconut
- 2 cups brown sugar
- 1/2 sticks butter, softened,
- 1 teaspoon baking powder
- 1 teaspoon baking soda
- 2 whole eggs
- 1 teaspoon vanilla
- 1 cup milk
- 2 1/4 cups flour
- ½ tsp cinnamon
- 1/2 teaspoon nutmeg.

Preheat oven 350 degrees F. In a mixing bowl, toss the mandarin orange with 1 cup of brown sugar, 1/2 teaspoon cinnamon, and 1/2 teaspoon nutmeg. Mix dry and wet ingredients to make cake mixture in a round cake pan place oranges around the edge put coconut mixture in the middle pour cake batter and bake 1 hour.

STEEL DRUMS

- 4-6 coconut halves
- 2 cup berries
- 1 cup mango
- 1 cup papaya
- ¼ cup guava paste or puree
- ¼ cup cream of coconut
- shredded coconut
- orange juice
- lemon juice
- lime juice

Marinate fruit in citrus juices for a few minutes to prevent them from turning brown and adds extra flavor stir in coconut milk, shredded coconut and guava paste into coconut cut in halves cover with foil

Place coconut halves in baking dish with water very low just for steaming steam bake bout half hour

SWEET PLANTAIN EMPANADA

- 3-4 sweet plantain or small brown ones
- empanada dough rounds
- ½ cup raisins
- rum optional
- peanut oil for frying
- veggie margarine or soy

Peel and cut plantain sauté in sauce pan with margarine

Add raisins rum if want place 2 or 3 spoonfuls of mixture in the empanada rounds fry on each side in peanut oil till lightly browned

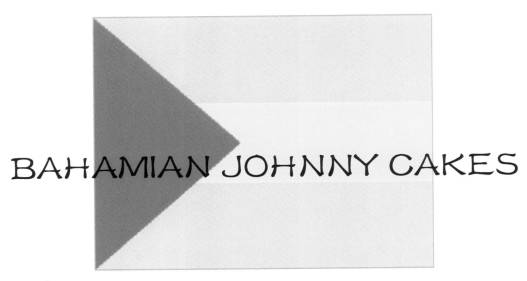

BAHAMIAN JOHNNY CAKES

- 1 egg, beaten
- 1 cup of milk
- 1 cup of flour
- 1/3 cup of sugar
- 3/4 cup of cornmeal
- 3/4 teaspoon of salt
- 5 teaspoons of baking powder
- 2 tablespoons vegetable oil

Preheat the oven to 350 F. Mix all of the dry ingredients together. Add egg, milk and oil to dry mixture and blend well. Pour into 8 inch square pan. Bake for 30 to 35 minutes until slightly brown On top. Serve hot or cold with butter, or honey.

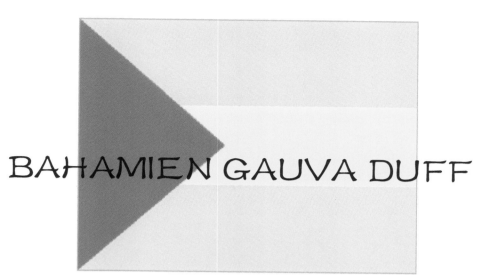

BAHAMIEN GAUVA DUFF

- 4 cups flour,
- 1 cup sugar,
- 1 ½ tsp baking powder,
- 1 tsp salt,
- ½ cup vegetable oil,
- 2 cups finely sliced guava

Combine all dry ingredients and mix together. Add oil. Knead approximately 10 minutes until smooth and pliable. Place on a flat surface and roll out to ¼ in. thick. Spread sliced guava over dough. Roll up into a long round loaf. Wrap in foil. Cook in a double boiler for 1 hr.

BIBLICAL CAKE

- 3 cups wheat flour
- 2 cups raw brown sugar
- 1 cup honey
- 1 cup sliced almonds
- 4 cups pomegranate juice
- 1 tsp cinnamon
- ½ cup extra virgin olive oil
- 1 cup figs (chopped)
- ½ cup dates(chopped)
- ½ cup water

Grease loaf pan and set aside. Soak chop figs and dates in 3 cups pomegranate juice

This can be done up to a 2 weeks ahead of time. Must be kept cool. In a mixing a bowl combine wheat flour, cinnamon and brown sugar. Add remaining pomegranate juice, olive oil and water. Mix until completely combined. Fold in fruit and honey then fold in almonds last. Pour batter in greased loaf pan and bake in oven for 45 minutes – 1 hour.

Test with bamboo stick.

Can refer to for ingredients Genesis, Exodus, Jeremiah, Samuel, and Numbers.

Breads and Pizzas

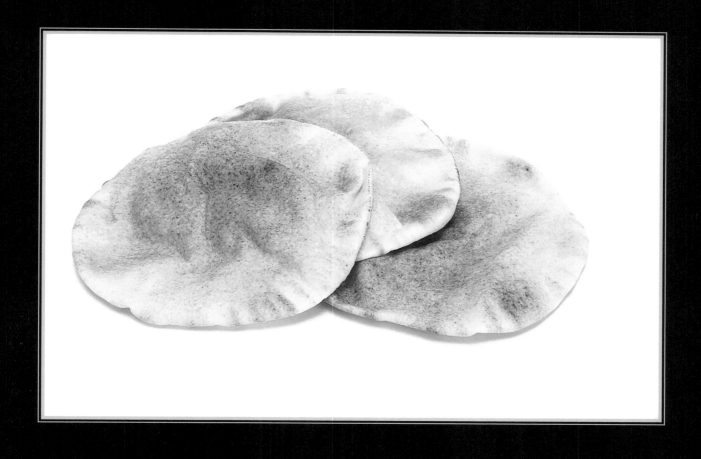

GRILLED VEGETABLE PIZZA

- Non-stick cooking spray
- 1 red onion (sliced)
- 4 plum tomatoes (sliced thin)
- 2 small Japanese egg plants (sliced)
- 1 zucchini (sliced)
- 2 cloves garlic (minced)
- 2 T parmesan cheese (optional)
- 1 T fresh basil (chopped)
- kosher salt and black pepper
- 1 large ready made pizza dough

Preheat broiler. Lightly grease baking sheet with non stick cooking spray. Place vegetables on sheet turning frequently, until browned. Spread tomatoes, basil and garlic evenly over pizza. Then top with broiled vegetables and cheese. Bake for 15 minutes. Season with salt and pepper.

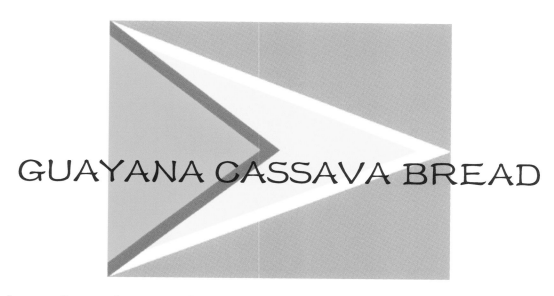

GUAYANA CASSAVA BREAD

Peel, wash and grate the cassava. Squeeze out as much of the juice as possible, using either a matapee or by wringing in a towel.

The juice can be used for making cassareep. Leave in lumps and allow to dry slightly in open air. Pound, sift and add salt.

Heat a griddle and a metal hoop of the size of cake required. Put enough of the cassava meal to a depth of about 1/8 to 1/4 inch in the hoop.

Cook until set, using moderate heat. Remove the hoops, level surface, press firmly. Turn onto the other side and cook.

When cooked through, remove the cake and sun dry till crisp.

HARD DOUGH BREAD

- 1 1/2 lbs. all-purpose flour
- 1/2 oz. fresh yeast OR 1 rounded tsp. dried yeast
- 2 tsp. salt
- 2 tbsp. vegetable shortening (optional)
- 1 tsp. granulated sugar
- 1/2 pint warm water
- 2 beaten egg whites OR milk, for brushing tops of loaves

Preheat oven to 350°F (180°C). It takes 40 minutes for the loaf to bake.

All ingredients and utensils should be warmed to assist the fermentation.

Dissolve the yeast in some of the liquid and add 1 teaspoon sugar. Leave it to stand in a warm place for 10 minutes. This activates the yeast and starts the fermentation process.

Sift the flour and salt together. (Rub in the 2 tbsp. shortening, if being used).

Add the yeast liquid and the rest of the liquid all at once.

Mix quickly to a soft dough which is elastic and pliable.

Knead the dough vigorously either by hand or in an electric mixer, using dough hook. Kneading ensures thorough distribution of yeast in the dough so that it is in contact with the natural sugars in the flour. It also helps to develop the gluten so that it is capable of stretching during fermentation.

Cover the dough with a damp cloth to prevent the formation of a skin and leave it to rise or 'proof' in a warm place for 1 to 2 hours. During this time the process of fermentation takes place. The temperature inside the dough should be about 77°F (25°C) to work efficiently.

Knock back (punch) the dough by kneading it again to bring the yeast into contact with more of the flour.

Shape the dough into loaves or rolls. Place in 9 x 5-inch greased loaf pans and leave to rise again for 40 minutes so that more Carbon Dioxide gas is produced.

Brush top of loaves with milk or beaten egg whites.

Bake at 350°F (180°C) for 30-40 minutes or until set and golden brown in color, and bottom sounds hollow when tapped

I-MAN BLACK BEAN PIZZA

- Flat bread or pita
- Cooked black beans (see below)
- 2 cloves garlic
- ½ cup chopped seeded tomato
- 1 T thyme
- ¼ cup chopped cilantro
- BEANS; cook beans
- Coconut milk
- Bell peppers
- Onion
- Thyme
- Cilantro
- Mashed garlic
- Scotch bonnet optional

Mash black beans in to a paste spread on bread and top with tomato or your favorite toppings bake till bubbly.

INJERA

- 3/4 cup teff, ground fine
- 3 1/2 cups water
- salt
- sunflower or other vegetable oil

Mix ground teff with 3 1/2 cups water and let stand in a bowl covered with a dish towel, at room temperature, until it bubbles and has turned sour. This may take as long as 3 days. The fermenting mixture should be the consistency of pancake batter (which is exactly what it is).Stir in salt, a little at a time, until you can barely detect the taste. Lightly oil your largest skillet. Heat over medium-high heat. Then proceed as you would with a normal pancake or crepe. Pour in enough batter to cover the bottom of the skillet. About 1/4 cup will make a thin pancake covering the surface of an 8-inch skillet if you spread the batter around immediately by turning and rotating the skillet in the air. This is the classic French method for very thin crepes. Injera is not supposed to be paper thin so you should use a bit more batter than you would for crepes, but less than you would for a flapjack. It should be about 1/3 inch thick. Cook briefly, until holes form in the injera and the edges lift from the pan. Remove and let cool

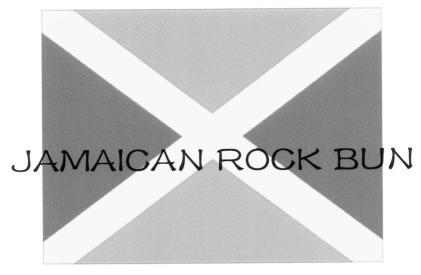

JAMAICAN ROCK BUN

- 1 large egg
- 8 ounces of flour
- 3 ounces of butter
- 4.5 ounces of sugar
- 4 ounces of raisins
- 3 ounces of butter
- 1 teaspoon vanilla,
- nutmeg and cinnamon
- 1 teaspoon of baking
- -powder

First combine together the butter and sugar. Add the beaten egg and vanilla.

Now stir into flour with baking powder along with the raisins and the spices.

Next roll into buns. Bake in a heated oven at 350 degrees F.

LIONESS TARTS

- Flat bread or pita
- Tomato paste or puree
- Sliced thin yellow bell pepper
- Sliced thin green bell pepper
- Sliced and seeded tomato
- Sliced pineapple
- Garlic powder

Mix garlic powder in paste spread evenly on bread, place peppers, toamtos and pineapple slices bake till bubbly

ROTI

- 1 cup of wheat flour
- 2 tablespoons of oil
- Salt and enough water
- -to make dough

Knead the wheat flour, salt and water to make dough. Let the dough stand for half hour.

Take small portions, knead again, and dust with the flour and roll out into a round shape.

Cook in (flat) griddle with a little oil (Flip on both sides can add vegetables

SUN DRIED TOMATO PIZZA

- Pita bread
- Tomatoes paste
- 1-2 garlic clove grated and mashed
- fresh basil
- 2 cup sun dried tomato

Mix in a bowl tomatoes paste and grated garlic till well blended spread on pita bread chop sun dried tomatoes and place on top of tomatoes paste add fresh basil and bake till bubbly and lightly browned

Soups and Stews

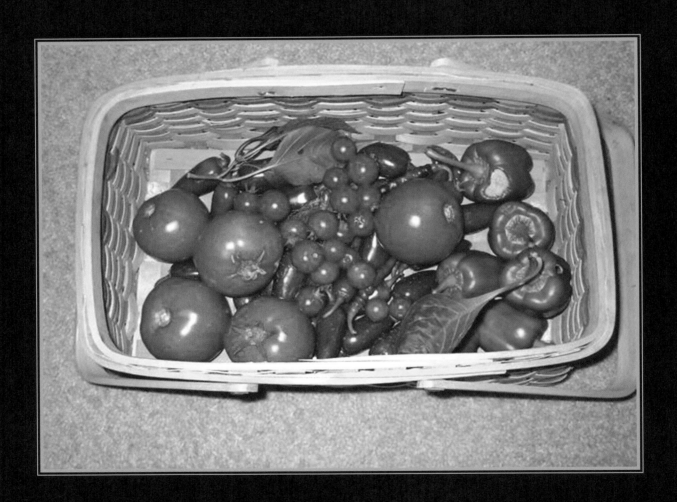

BLACK EYE PEA AND OKRA STEW

- 1 cup yellow onion, diced
- 2 cloves garlic, chopped
- 3 cups fresh okra, cut into rounds
- 2 cups fresh corn
- 1 scotch bonnet pepper, chopped
- 2 cups black-eyed peas
- 1 cup tomatoes (seeded and chopped)
- Salt
- Pepper
- Freshly chopped cilantro, for garnish
- 2 ½ cups vegetable broth

Rinse and soak black eye peas overnight. In a large pot, cover peas with veggie broth. Bring to a boil and add all remaining ingredients. Cook until peas are tender. Serve with rice.

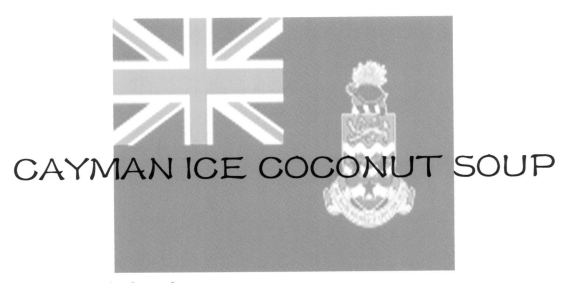

CAYMAN ICE COCONUT SOUP

- 1 cup veggie broth
- 1 can of 14 oz. coconut milk
- - (not sweetened as for drinks)
- 2 teaspoons pepper & salt
- curry powder for flavor

First in a blender add all of the ingredients

Now chill the coconut soup in the frigerator.

Serve this delicious soup with slices of cold honeydew melon

MOCK COCK SOUP

- 1 cup chopped yellow onion
- 1 cup chopped yellow bell pepper
- ½ cup chopped scallion
- 1 cup thin sliced carrot
- 2 cup cut potato
- 1 cup thin whole wheat spaghetti broke in 1 inch pieces
- ½ cup green peas
- 1 T curry powder
- 1tsp dried thyme
- 1tsp ground ginger
- 1 orange scotch bonnet
- 4 cups veggie broth
- water

In a soup pot brown the onions, peppers and seasonings, add 4 cups vegetable broth and water. Add potatoes, peas and carrots bring to boil and add spaghetti cook till potatoes and spaghetti is tender serve with flat bread

CURRY CORN SOUP

- 1lb corn (frozen or cobbed) (plus cobbed corn cut into rounds)
- 2 onions (coarsely chopped)
- 2 cloves garlic (minced)
- 1 green pepper (coarsely chopped)
- ½ cup tomatoes (chopped & seeded)
- 1 pkg. (GOYA) sazon
- 4 tsp chili powder
- 4 T curry powder
- 2 T butter or 3 T olive oil
- 4 cups vegetable stock or water
- 1 cup coconut milk
- salt & black pepper if desired
- more water if needed
- chopped cilantro (for garnish)

Sautee onions, garlic, bell pepper and tomato in stock pot with butter or olive oil. Stir in sazon, chili powder and curry, brown veggies in seasonings. Then add coconut milk and vegetable stock or water. Cut corn into rounds and add your 1lb of corn and the corn rounds. Stir occasionally, bring to a boil. Cook about 20 minutes.

EAST AFRICAN SWEET PEA SOUP

- 2 cups chopped onion
- 2 tsp minced garlic
- 1 tsp grated fresh peeled ginger
- 1 tsp salt
- 1/4 tsp cayenne pepper
- 1 tbsp homemade garam masala
- 1/2 tsp ground black pepper
- 1 tsp ground coriander seeds

- 1 tsp ground cumin seeds
- 1/4 tsp ground cardamom
- 1/8 tsp ground cloves
- 1/4 tsp cinnamon
- 1 tsp turmeric
- 2 tomatoes, chopped
- 1 sweet potato, diced
- 3 1/2 cups water
- 3 cups fresh green peas

Braise/deglaze onions and garlic in a pot for 5-10 minutes.

Mix in the ginger, salt, and all spices and cook for a few minutes, stirring often.

Add tomatoes and sweet potato, stir. Add 1 1/2 cups of water, stir.

Bring soup to a boil, reduce heat, cover, and simmer for 5 minutes.

Add 2 cups of the peas and simmer, covered, for 10 minutes.

Remove from heat and add remaining 2 cups of water. Puree in batches in a blender until smooth. Return to the pot, add the last cup of peas, and cook on medium heat for 3-5 minute

ITAL STEW

- 1 hot pepper
- 1 pound of yam
- 1 pound of coco
- 3 green bananas juice of 1/2 lime
- 1 pound of pumpkin
- 1/2 pound of cassava
- 1/2 pound of breadfruit
- 2 pints of vegetable stock
- freshly ground black pepper
- plain or cornmeal dumplings
- 1/2 cup of coconut milk

First you must remove the seeds from the pumpkin. Wash and peel the yam, pumpkin, coco and the cassava.

Next slice breadfruit in wedges, peel and cut out the heart. Chop all the vegetable In fairly large pieces.

Now bring the stock to a boil in a large Pan. Add vegetables, hot pepper with the black pepper. Turn heat down then simmer for about 20 minutes.

Mix the dumplings and add to the pan, turn up the heat and cook it till the dumplings are done.

In a separate pan boil the green bananas in their skins, having cut off both ends split The skin deeply with a knife.

When cooked, allow to cool a little before peeling. Cut each banana into 3 pieces and add to the stew with the lime juice.

Finally, remove the hot pepper once the stew has been reheated.

JAMAICAN COLD ALVOCODO SOUP

- 1/4 cup butter
- 1 cup finely chopped onion
- 2 1/2 teaspoons fresh ginger, peeled and grated (about 1 ounce)
- 2 large ripe avocados, peeled and mashed

- 4 teaspoons fresh lime juice
- 1 1/2 cups veggie stock
- 1/2 teaspoon black pepper
- 1 green onion, finely chopped
- 1/2 cup half-and-half
- Salt and freshly grated black pepper

Lime Crema:
- 1/4 cup sour cream
- 2 teaspoons fresh lime juice
- 1/4 teaspoon minced garlic

Melt the butter in a saucepan and cook the onions for about 4 minutes, until softened. Add the ginger and continue to cook an additional 2 minutes. Add the avocado, lime juice, and veggie stock and whisk to combine. Simmer soup over medium-low heat for about 5 minutes. Add the green onion and transfer the soup to a blender and puree, in batches if necessary, until very smooth. Stir in the half-and-half and pepper, to taste. Chill thoroughly before serving.

To make the lime crema, stir together the sour cream, lime juice, garlic, when the soup has chilled, garnish each portion with a generous dollop of cream. Salt if desired (kosher)

PASSION SOUP

- 2 Passion Fruits
- 2 vanilla bean pods
- 1/2 cored pineapple - chopped
- 1 papaya - peeled and chopped
- 1 mango -peeled and chopped
- 3 cups cubed watermelon
- 1 cup of coconut milk
- 1/2 cup cream of coconut
- 1 teaspoon nutmeg

Cut passion fruits in half and scoop out the seeds and throw them away. Squeeze the passion fruit into a strainer and save the juice. Cut the vanilla bean pods in half length wise and take out the seeds and set them aside.

In a food processor, combine half the passion fruit juice and the vanilla seeds. Add half the pineapple, papaya, mango, watermelon, coconut milk and coconut cream. Blend until smooth.

Place mixture in a large bowl and repeat the process with the remaining ingredients.

Lastly, stir in the nutmeg and garnish with toasted coconut. Refrigerate for about an hour

PEANUT SOUP

- 2 large sweet potatoes (about 2 pounds)
- 4 tablespoons peanut oil
- 12 Roma plum tomatoes, halved, stems removed and seeded (about 2 pounds)
- 1/2 teaspoon ground black pepper
- 2 tablespoons curry powder
- 2 cups thinly sliced yellow onions
- 1 tablespoon minced garlic
- 2 teaspoons cayenne pepper
- 2 cups smooth peanut butter
- 2 quarts veggie broth
- 10 ounces unsweetened coconut milk

Preheat oven to 375 degrees F.

Lightly coat the sweet potatoes with 1 tablespoon of the oil. Place on a baking sheet and roast until fork tender, turning once, 35 to 45 minutes. Toss the tomato halves with 1 tablespoon of the oil and spread in 1 layer on a baking sheet. Lightly season with pepper, and bake until shriveled, 20 minutes. Remove both the potatoes and tomatoes from the oven. Peel the potatoes when cool enough to handle.

Heat the remaining 2 tablespoons of oil in a small stockpot over medium-high heat. Add the curry powder and toast until aromatic, stirring constantly, for 2 minutes. Add the onions and cook until soft, 3 minutes. Add the garlic, and cook, stirring, for 30 seconds. Season with the cayenne, then add the peanut butter, and stir well. Add the tomatoes, peeled potatoes, veggie stock, and coconut milk and bring to a boil. Reduce the heat to medium-low and simmer for 15 minutes. Salt if desired (kosher) Salt if desired (kosher)

PLANTAIN PORRIDGE

- 4 cups water
- 6 green bananas (medium size)
- Salt and pepper to taste

Put 2 cups water in saucepan to boil.

Peel bananas and blender with two cups of water and salt until the desired consistency is reached. Pour the blend in the boiling water and stir until bananas are cooked

POTATO SOUP

- 3 cups cut potato
- ½ cup chopped carrots
- 2-3 stalks celery chopped
- ¼ cup chopped onion
- ¼ cup chopped red bell pepper
- 2 cloves mashed garlic
- 1 T parsley
- 1T chopped chives
- 2 cups broccoli florets
- 1 cup chop cauliflower
- veggie broth
- salt and white pepper if desired

Cook potato in veggie broth and mashed garlic till done, taking half potatoes out of pot puree and return to soup add remaining ingredients cook till tender

RAW CUCUMBER CARROT SOUP

- whole cucumber
- carrots
- ½ onion
- 1 stalk celery for seasoning
- 1 tsp lime juice
- 1pine apple juice
- cilantro for garnish

- In a juicer add carrots, cucumber, onion and celery. Squeeze lime pine apple juice, in juices stir and chill
- Garnish with fresh cut cilantro when served.
-

ROCKERS STEW

- 1 cup potato
- 1 cup yellow yam
- 1 cup sweet potato
- ½ cup chopped onion
- ½ cup chopped scallions
- ½ cup chopped green bell pepper
- ½ cup chopped carrots
- 2 green plantain
- ½ cup cassava (yucca)
- 1T dried thyme
- 1T cilantro
- 2 cloves garlic
- ½ tsp lemon zest
- scotch bonnet (optional)
- 4 cups veggie broth
- water if needed

Peel potatoes, yams and cut in cubes, chop and mash garlic

(Try hand grater) for garlic

Sauté onions and peppers till lightly brown add veggie broth and bring to boil. Add potato and yams and seasonings... add lemon zest at this time; cook till all is tender   save some chopped fresh cilantro to sprinkle on top.

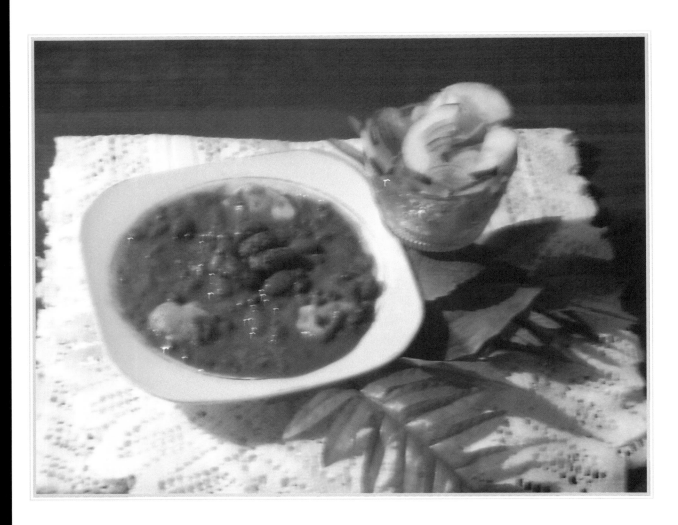

SPICY STEW BEANS & DUMPLINGS

- 2 cans of red beans
- 1 whole scotch bonnet
- 3 whole stalk escallion
- dried whole leaf thyme
- 1/2 of block of cooking butter
- 1/4 ounces of green seasoning in bottle
- 2 packs of sazon accent
- 1 can of coconut milk

Melt the butter. Combine all ingredients together sauté seasonings and peas then cover with water add coconut milk and scotch bonnet once beans are tender add cooked dumplings and let simmer remove whole scotch bonnet

DUMPLINS:
- 2 cups flour
- 2 tsp baking powder
- 1/2 tsp salt
- 1 cup water or milk to bind flour
- cooking oil to fry

Mix flour baking powder and salt in a medium bowl with a whisk. Bind the flour with warm water or milk When it comes together remove bowl and knead.

If preparing for soup or stew, spoonfuls can be dropped for 15-20 minutes (stop here)! If frying, divide dough in 2, roll into a 6x2 inch shape. Put on a cutting board and cut in 1/2 inch diagonals. Heat enough oil to deep fry, about 5 mins. per side till golden

SUNSET SOUP

YELLOW SPLIT PEA ROASTED BELL PEPPER)

- 1 Bag dried yellow split peas
- 1 Cup yellow onion (chopped)
- 1 Cup roasted red bell pepper (chopped)
- ½ Cup celery (chopped)
- 1t dried parsely
- 1t dried thyme
- 2t curry powder
- 2t paprika
- 1t corriander powder
- 1ts ground ginger
- 1ts cumin
- 2 Cups vegetable broth
- Water
- Salt if desired
- 3 Cloves garlic (minced)
- Juice of half lemon

Clean, rinse and soak peas over night. Cover peas in soup pot about 3 inch above peas.

Add chopped vegetables and dried seasonings. Cook till tender and smooth. Mash and mix peas add more water if needed. Soup should be on the thin. Fold in roasted red bell pepper and juice of a half of lemon last twenty minutes of cooking.

VEGETABLE RUN DOWN

- 1 Cup veggie broth
- 4 Sprigs of Thyme
- 2 Garlic cloves, crushed
- 1 Large Onion, chopped fine
- 2 Large Tomatoes, chopped fine
- 2 cups cubed potato
- 1 cup chopped carrots
- 1-2 green plantain
- 2 Stalks of Escallion, chopped fine
- 2 Cups Coconut Milk or 1 Can Coconut Milk
- 1 Scotch Bonnet Pepper, chopped fine (Optional)

Sauté onions, scallion and peppers add tomatoe, carrots, plantain and potatoes add broth and seasonings steam down till done add coconut milk serve with roasted bread fruit

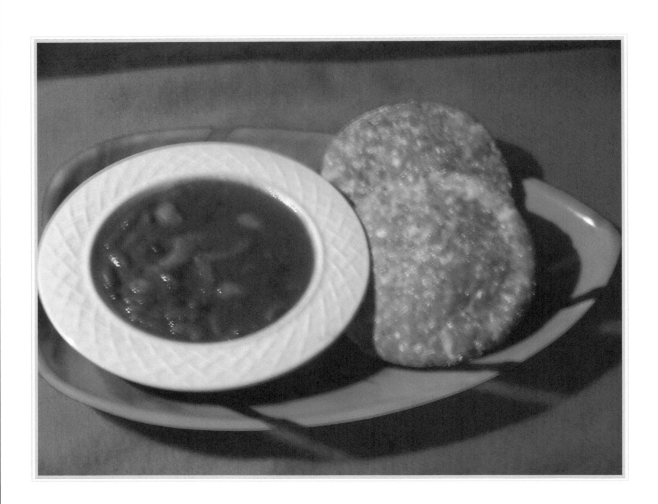

VEGETARIAN CHILI

- 1 bag red kidney bean
- 1 bag pink bean
- 2 cups black bean
- 2 cups lima bean
- 2 cup zucchini
- 2 cup yellow squash
- ½ cup chopped onion
- ½ cup chopped green bell pepper
- 1 cup seeded chopped tomatoes
- 3 cup tomatoes sauce
- ½-1 - tsp cayenne pepper
- 1 T chili powder
- veggie broth

Sauté onions and peppers, add beans. Cook beans till tender drain most water and adds veggie broth and chopped veggies add seasonings cook till all veggies and beans are tender make spicy as want

YUCCA VEGETABLE CHILI

- 11/4lb yucca cut into 1- inch chunks (peeled)
- 1 onion (chopped)
- 3 cloves garlic (minced)
- ½ red bell pepper & ½ green bell pepper
- 1 jalapeno (seeded & chopped)
- 1 16 oz can chickpeas (rinsed)
- 6 ripe tomatoes (peeled, seeded & chopped)
- 2 whole scallions (chopped)
- 1T cumin
- 1T ground coriander
- 2T chili powder
- juice of ½ lime
- 1 small bunch of cilantro (chopped)
- ½ cup grated cheddar cheese (optional)

Place yucca in a medium saucepan with salted water to cover. Squeeze the juice from the lime and add to the yucca. Simmer until tender, about 30 to 45 minutes. Meanwhile, in a large pot over medium heat, cook the onions, garlic, jalapenos, and bell pepper in margarine with the cumin, chili powder and ground coriander. Add chickpeas and tomatoes, and cook 3 minutes. Drain the yucca and add to the vegetable mixture. Cook until flavors are blended about 10 minutes. Before serving scatter scallions, cilantro and cheese (optional) over chili.

DRINKS AND BEVERAGES

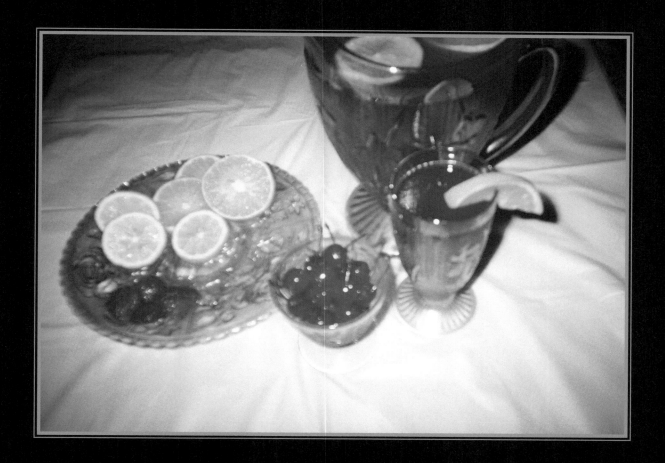

TEA, TEA

- 1cup brewed hibiscus tea
- 1 cup brewed raspberry tea
- 1 cup brewed white tea
- ½ cup natural brown sugar
- 1 qt. water

Mix all brewed teas in a pitcher with ice and sugar let chill serve with fresh mint and slice of fruit

BEETROOT DRINK

- 2 cups beetroot
- 1-2 celery stalk
- 1 lemon /lime
- 2 cups water
- 2 cups sugar

Wash beet and cut up coarsely. Extract juice from lemon/lime.

Boil beet and celery in water for 20 minutes, then strain. Stir sugar into the strained liquid, and then add lime/lemon juice.

Then pour into bottle. Leave to ferment for three weeks

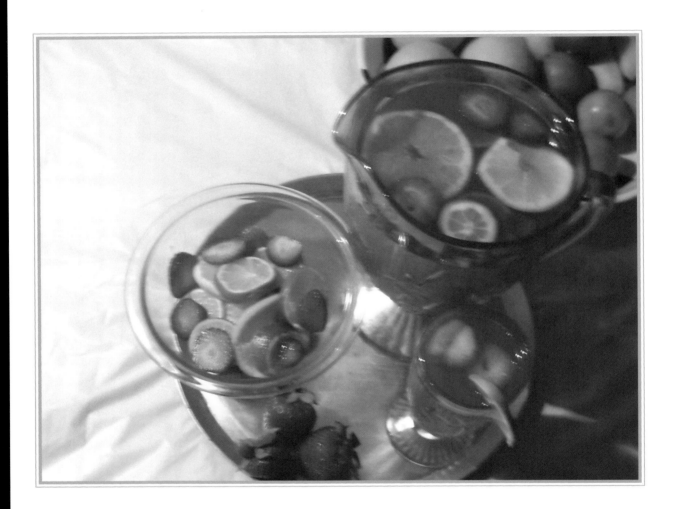

ETHIOPIAN PUNCH

- 1 cup raspberry syrup
- 1 cup maraschino cherry syrup
- 1cup orange juice
- 1 cup lemon juice
- 1 cup pineapple juice
- 1 cup grape juice
- 2-1/2 quarts

Mix in punch bowl garnish with fruit slices

GINGER BEER

- 1 gallon of water
- 2 ounces of ginger
- 5 to 6 heaped tablespoons of sugar

Grate the ginger and allow it to set in the water for about 1 day.

Strain and sweeten.

Or Combine two tablespoons of the ginger beer syrup along with 4 to 5 heaped tablespoons of sugar and 8 cups of water in a jar.

GUAVA LAVA

- 12 oz guava puree
- ¼ cup sweet milk
- ¼ cup strawberry syrup
- 20oz sparkling water

Blend puree sweet milk and syrup till well blended add sparkling water, ice and blend served chilled

LEMONGINGER AIDE

- 3 lemons cut and juiced
- 2 cups graded mashed ginger
- 2-1/2 quarts water
- ½ cup raw brown sugar

In a large pitcher mix lemon juice and sugar in a separate bowl soak ginger for ½ hour strain add ginger flavored water to pitcher stir served chilled with lemon wedge

MANGO SUNRISE PUNCH

- 1cup mango puree
- 20oz pomegranate juice
- 8oz sparkling water
- 1 orange for garnish

Blend juice and puree add sparkling water after blended garnish with orange slices

MAUBY

- 4 to 5 heaped tablespoons of sugar
- 2 ounces of mauby bark

Boil the mauby bark in 3 pints of the water until about 2/3 of the water has boiled off. The pint of mauby bitters must be refrigerated for future use.

Combine 1 to 2 teaspoons of the mauby bitters with the sugar and 8 ounces of water in a jar or you can combine 1 to 2 tablespoons of mauby syrup with 4 to 5 heaped tablespoons of sugar 8 cups of water.

MOUNTAIN MAN

- 1 cup coconut milk
- ½ cup papaya puree
- ½ cup mango juice
- 1 cup pineapple juice
- ½ tsp fresh ground nutmeg

Blend or shake the coconut milk, papaya puree adding the juices pineapple and mango after completely blended sprinkle nutmeg on top served chilled or warm

PINEAPPLE CARROT JAMMIE

- 20oz pineapple juice
- 12 0z carrot juice
- 8oz mineral water
- 1T lime juice

Mix juices, and tsp of fresh lime and shake with ice drain juice in glasses with out ice garnish with sliced lime

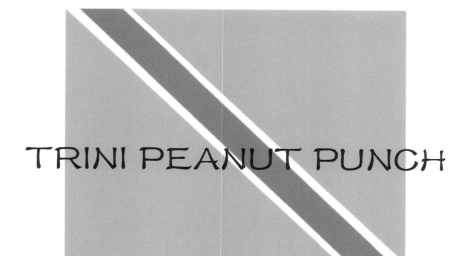

TRINI PEANUT PUNCH

- ½ cup of sugar
- 1 teaspoon of cinnamon
- 1/2 teaspoon of nutmeg
- 2 1/2 teaspoons peanut butter
- 1 qt. milk or soy milk

Blend together the milk, with the peanut butter along with sugar for about 3 to 4 minutes.

Next add the nutmeg and cinnamon to taste place the punch into the fridge chill and serve.

MENUS

EMPEROR'S EARTH DAY
(BIRTHDAY)

- King's Rice Salad
- Eggplant Rounds
- Carribean Corn On The Cob
- Mountain Man Drink
- Steel Drums

EMPRESS EARTH DAY
(BIRTHDAY)

- Empress Salad
- Bajan Black Beans & Mango Salsa
- I-N-I Tarts
- Tea, Tea

KIDS DAY

- Rasta Baby Logs
- Raga Raga Chips
- Warm Breeze Saghetti
- Guava Lava

SUNDAY BEST

- Ethiopian Toss
- Rockers Stew
- Coco Rice
- Injera
- Biblical Cake
- Ethiopian Punch

Printed in the United States
150638LV00003B